CAREGIVERS
Are People Too

A Primer for Those Who Take
Care of Disabled Persons

by
Gloria M. Sprung M.S.W.

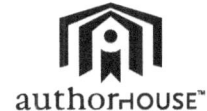

authorHOUSE™

1663 LIBERTY DRIVE, SUITE 200
BLOOMINGTON, INDIANA 47403
(800) 839-8640
WWW.AUTHORHOUSE.COM

First published by AuthorHouse 12/06/05

ISBN: 1-4208-7464-0 (sc)

Printed in the United States of America
Bloomington, Indiana

This book is printed on acid-free paper.

DISCLAIMER:

This book is based on the experiences of the author as a social worker and a caregiver. It is meant to help caregivers obtain a fuller life for themselves and their care recipients. It is not designed to take the place of your health professional. Your health professional and the health professional of your partner must be consulted before implementing any of the techniques described. It is essential that you discuss these techniques with your doctor and/or therapist, as the author is not responsible for any harmful results that may occur.

All the vignettes in this book are stories based on my many years of experience as a social worker, speech therapist, and teacher. The people depicted in the vignettes are not actual persons, but are products of the author's imagination. The events described are illustrative of situations that may occur, but all have no existence except in the author's mind. Any resemblance to actual people or events is purely coincidental.

The purpose of this book is to educate and encourage change. The author and publisher shall have neither liability nor responsibility to any person or entity with respect to any damage alleged to have been caused, directly or indirectly, by the information contained in this book.

Acknowledgments

This book was an outcome of a conversation I had with a psychiatrist who was a dear friend of mine. At that time I was working as a social worker and simultaneously serving as an active caregiver for a seriously handicapped stroke victim. I realized that the caregiving was consuming me and I was in the process of reassessing the situation and my role. While talking about my struggle, we decided that a book about caregiving could help other people mired in this task. Our idea was to help them examine their own motivations, and by so doing, enable them to climb out of this rut. Unfortunately, he died an untimely death soon after we discussed this project. I placed the idea for the book on the back burner for many years until I was encouraged to write it by another psychiatrist, Dr. David Pelino. He read my chapters as I developed them, and urged me to continue. I have known Dr. Pelino for twelve years, and he was of inestimable value in helping me cope with my own caregiving life, the anguish of the eventual nursing home placement and death of my husband.

This book is not intended to be an expert analysis of the various handicapping conditions discussed in the second section. The conditions are discussed in generalities and are geared to help the caregiver climb out of his self-defeating life and hopefully find a new approach that will help him embark on a happier, more self-satisfying life. It is also hoped that by doing that, his partner will be encouraged to find a better style of life despite his disabilities, rather than live an unfulfilling one because of them. It is not intended as a reference book, only as a guide for caregivers. The suggestions of behavior modification should be discussed with your partner's therapist or physician before being implemented, to prevent any unforeseen results.

This book reflects the soul-searching struggles I had defining and re-defining myself through many difficult years. My hope is that the reader will be encouraged to do the same.

I want to dedicate this book to the memory of my husband. Helping him survive the residual damage of his stroke humbled me as well as taught me how to face the changes in his life and mine. I also dedicate it to our daughter, Geri, whose love and devotion were of inestimable value and a bulwark of strength for me during these difficult times.

I offer sincere thanks to Dr. Pelino for his friendship and his encouragement. Without that, I would have never "birthed" this book.

Gloria Sprung

Foreword

The nuclear age and the scientific era have had an impact not only on economics and world-shaking politics but also upon the individual's daily life. Modern medicine has prolonged life, enabled mental patients to leave the state hospitals, and turned formerly terminal illnesses into chronic debilitating conditions. Thus, we have many more people who are living outside of institutions and hospitals, fraught with problems of significant magnitude – problems of a physical nature and/or mental disorders. Many other people are affected by these phenomena – particularly those who share their home and their lives with relatives who are mentally disabled, brain injured or otherwise physically incapacitated (on dialysis, in chronic pain, paraplegic etc.)

In the literature, this type of couple is often referred to as the caregiver and the caretaker. That, in turn, implies one passive person and one active one. If the situation is seen in this way, both parties eventually find they become angry, hostile, bitter, and frustrated. What we have are a minimum of two people, one who has a condition which creates innumerable problems in daily living, and another who, for whatever motives, has chosen to share his life with this chronically impaired individual. Many caregivers at this point will jump up indignantly and say there was no choice. "I had to do it – no other way, no money, no one else."

The basic tenet of this book is that there is always a choice. If you can accept this premise, there is reason to hope, and with hope comes better ways of coping with different problems. When one is forced to live with another whose life is filled with physical or mental obstacles, one may become a part of the problem, remain apart from the problem, or become a partner in coping with the problem.

This is not a manual for surviving with schizophrenia or bearing with brain damage or dealing with dialysis. These conditions are difficult and heartrending, and each presents its own particular problems. It is certainly important to see that aspect. But in a more generic sense, there are coping mechanisms which can be sharpened and strengthened, and allow families to live a fuller and happier life, even though it must be shared with a difficult and often heart-rending situation.

Table of Contents

Section One: Self-Assessment for a New Perspective

Chapter 1
Wilt with Guilt   3

Chapter 2
Buying the Ticket   12

Chapter 3
Sin of Kin   18

Chapter 4
Use of Abuse   27

Chapter 5
The Parasite's Might   38

Chapter 6
The Right of Fight   45

Chapter 7
Moving On   52

Section Two: Defining His Issues; Redefining Yours

Chapter 8
Living with Mental Illness   65

Chapter 9
Living With the Frail Elderly   78

Chapter 10
Living with a Mentally Challenged Person   91

Chapter 11
Living With a Physically Ill Person   98

Chapter 12
Living With an Addicted Person   106

Section Three: Considering Alternatives

Chapter 13
Be Fair to Homecare   115

Chapter 14
What About Day Care?   121

Chapter 15
Working for the Disabled   127

Chapter 16
Journey's End   133

Section One:
Self-Assessment for a New Perspective

Chapter 1
Wilt with Guilt

Getting started on a journey is very different for different people. Some move slowly and carefully in an organized fashion, planning each step, researching stops, creating timetables, learning about all the attractions, and attempting to avoid pitfalls. Thus, by the time they buy their ticket, they know exactly where they want to go, how long they want to stay, and when they will be ready to leave. Others are much more haphazard. They decide they want to go somewhere, pick a few places, get a smattering of advice from friends and neighbors, and go buy their ticket. They have only a vague notion of how long they will stay anywhere but are fairly sure of where they are going. Still others are impetuous, deciding to go on a trip next week, picking a destination and planning to take it day by day.

How does this relate to your care giving situation and what I term the Samaritan Syndrome? Well, whether you go on a trip to an exotic foreign country or embark on a journey of living, you behave in your own characteristic fashion. If the journey goes on long enough, you may even forget why you decided to take it or how it happened that you started in New York and are now trekking through the Sahara.

The trip we are going to discuss is the journey you have chosen to take with another person. (I will use the masculine pronoun throughout this book for simplicity's sake. Naturally, women are prone to the same conditions and dynamics as their male counterparts.) The other person is handicapped and faces multiple problems of living. He might be elderly, struggling with the infirmities of old age, or mentally retarded, or addicted to drugs or alcohol, or suffering from severe emotional problems, or afflicted with a physical disease that severely limits his or her ability to take care of himself. You have chosen to share your life with this person who, in all probability, is related to you — a spouse, a parent, a child, a sibling, or a significant other.

Because you have been on this journey of caring for someone else for such a long time, by now you have probably forgotten how this trip began, or more importantly, why you chose to take it. If someone asked, you might answer, "I had no choice! What did you expect me to do, toss her out in the street? Let her rot and suffer? Who else was going to provide the care if I didn't? The Sandman? The Tooth Fairy? I tell you, I had no choice!"

These answers come quickly and glibly, especially when you feel you have to excuse or defend your position. However, right now, as you sit here reading this chapter, "someone else" is not asking you how or when you began this one-way trip of sacrificing your life to care for another. Instead, you are asking the questions, and since no one else is going to hear your answers, you have an opportunity to be completely truthful and not censor your thoughts or feelings, no matter how nasty or unspeakable they may be. In being so refreshingly honest with yourself, you will arrive at some fresh answers to problems that have long since gone stale.

With this in mind, let's start again. How did it happen that you started taking care of someone who could no longer manage on his or her own? Think back for a minute. By now, the beginning is somewhat a blur and no doubt full of painful memories.

Perhaps it began when you noticed your elderly mother was becoming for-getful. She rambled on and on about the past, but could not remember where she put her glasses or her keys. Then there was that funny time she put the ice cream in the closet instead of the freezer; and that not-so-funny time when she left the gas stove burner on all night. Something had to be done and you just had to do it.

Or perhaps it began shortly after your son was born. He did not look like your other children, that was true, but he was a sweet boy who never cried much or fussed and seemed perfectly okay — just different. Then you noticed that at nine months, he still could not crawl or even sit up by himself. The pediatrician, when asked face-to-face what was the problem, averted his eyes and mumbled that your boy was retarded, and sent you to a specialist. He con-firmed the fact that he was severely retarded and someone would need to care for him the rest of his life. So you devoted yourself to the task.

Or perhaps it began more gradually. Your husband had lost another job. His gambling problem seemed a little better but the drinking had gotten worse. The kids went their way and stayed out of his. You were doing all you could to keep him from skidding into skid row, where all the skidding stops. You worked with him, fought with him, and talked with him endlessly and futilely about his drinking. Then there was the night he came home even later, even more drunk, and your confrontation led to a rage that destroyed the clock on the mantle and destroyed you as well. You decided that would be the last fight. To keep the peace, there would be no more fuss. Someone had to take care of him, so you accepted the responsibility.

Or perhaps it began more like a dream that turned into a nightmare. Your daughter had always been so sensitive, so imaginative, but never sad or withdrawn — or at least not till high school. Then she stopped going out and stayed in her room. She stopped eating meals with the family and let her studies slip and thought about God-knows-what, until that awful night: the overdose of sleeping pills, the emergency room, the brief psychiatric hospitalization. Later, the longer stay at the state hospital and the diagnosis – chronic undifferentiated schizophrenia. Someone needed to take care of her and you knew it had to be you.

Or perhaps it began all at once. You were at the office. The house was paid for and the kids had finished their education. Despite your differences with your wife over the years, you and she were finally settling into the twilight years. Then the phone call came from the hospital and that first frightful visit to her bedside in the intensive care unit. In the morning, you had said goodbye to her as she was cleaning up the breakfast dishes, and in the afternoon — after the stroke, the call to 911, the ambulance, the hospital admission, you were looking at a paralyzed woman. Someone was going to need to take care of her and you promised "in sickness and in health."

Of course, you have your own individual scenario of how your trip began. But after the period of numbness passed, you probably can recall that you asked "Why did this happen?" To that question, a professional may have given you an answer, or at least a partial answer. "Loss of memory and confusion happens to a lot of people as they get old; some people are far more afflicted then others." Or, "Schizophrenia is caused by a biochemical imbalance we are trying to understand." or, "Alcoholism is a poorly understood illness which causes some people to be unusually susceptible to dependency on the drug." Or, "Mental retardation is generally regarded as just one of many birth defects that are could be genetically determined." Or "Your wife's cerebral vascular accident was caused by a combination of arteriosclerosis and hypertension."

These answers fall short of the mark. They describe <u>what</u> happened; they don't tell you how to deal with it. Sure, you now had an explanation or at least a label, Alzheimer's, bipolar affective illness, Down's syndrome, substance abuse disorder, renal insufficiency. These explanations appease our intellectual need to understand what went awry. As you think back, you'll recall that these explanations were not very comforting, because you were not simply interested in "Why did this happen?" What you also wanted to know was "Why did this happen to *him* and what will it mean to *me*?"

By now, you may have forgotten that you ever asked yourself such a question and even at the time, you may have posed the question in such a soft whisper that you barely heard yourself ask it. But we promise you, if you are now locked into the Samaritan Syndrome, at some point along the way, you asked yourself "What did **I do to deserve this**?" It is that kind of question — not the event itself — that led to your buying a ticket for the guilt trip you are now taking.

The question "Why did this happen to me?" is not such a bad one. In fact, there are really no such things as bad questions — just bad answers. So the problem is not that you wondered why you were placed in the position of caregiver. The problem is that you did not come up with a reasonable answer. Let's look at some of the possible answers you chose.

Mary is a sweet gal. (Everyone thinks so but Mary.) As she was growing up, what she lacked in love, she made up for with her imagination. As a kid, while her parents were screaming at each other about money or extramarital affairs or selfish in-laws, Mary would stay off in a corner and privately use her imagination to protect her from the family's version of acid rain. She would imagine that both her parents would be killed in a car accident and her nice aunt from Iowa would come and take her to the farm, where Mary would frolic in the wheat fields and marry a man who raised crops and not his voice. But Mary's imagination, powerful as it was, could not make the wish come true. As her feelings towards her parents became more bitter, her wish that her father would "drop dead" became more entrenched.

By the time Mary was in high school, the wishes were no longer conscious. Then one day it happened. She walked into her house after school and was greeted by her tearful mother and the news that her father had indeed dropped dead of a heart attack at work. No one was surprised that Mary helped her fragile mother get through the funeral and the painful grieving period but when sweet Mary quit high school to devote her entire life to consoling and caring for her mother, people wondered if Mary's behavior might not be somewhat extreme. But Mary saw it as her duty. For reasons outside her awareness, she felt obligated to remain the devoted daughter, doting on her mother night and day. Mary did not realize that her Samaritan Syndrome was an attempt to undo guilt. Her wish had come true, at least the part of the wish that wanted her father to drop dead.

Mary's case is more straightforward than most. Usually the anger is better disguised and the caregiver is even less aware that the extreme sacrifices for another actually derive from an attempt to undo angry wishes.

Joe is a good example. Joe had been dumped by his first love and married his wife to "get even." He never loved his wife much in the first place and loved her even less after they discovered she had a progressive neurological disease. He felt sorry for her, but could never admit to himself, and certainly not admit to his wife, that he was angry about her incessant demands. When she complained about the lumpy mattress or cold breakfast in bed, Joe never acknowledged to himself that he wished the whiny bitch would croak. Instead, he tried even more desperately to undo the guilt that derived from this hidden wish and strived every day harder and harder to please the woman he resented.

The point of these examples is that if Mary or Joe had honestly asked himself or herself the question "What did I do to deserve this?" They would have admitted that they believed they were being punished because their angry wishes had come true. They got trapped into the Samaritan Syndrome because they did not realize that their devoted care did not stem from true love but rather from a guilt that wouldn't go away no matter how hard they tried to care.

Sometimes this dynamic is subtler. Betsy, a thirty-year-old secretary, called off her wedding and quit her job so that she could care for her father, who had become bedridden after a severe heart attack. Betsy was convinced that her father's heart attack had been caused because the day before she had had a major argument with him about her coming marriage and his future son-in-law. They both became extremely agitated and she had stormed out of the house. In Betsy's mind, her father's heart attack was caused by the strain she had put on him by arguing so vehemently. It was all her fault. This belief was what led Betsy to buy a ticket on the guilt trip.

Jenny ended up being taken for the same kind of ride. Jenny believed her child was schizophrenic because she had gotten drunk at a party when she was pregnant, despite her doctor's orders not to drink. Jenny would do anything for her son (except set firm limits) to atone for the crime that she had committed. Jenny allowed her schizophrenic son behave anyway he saw fit. As a result as he became older and stronger his outrageous acts became more dangerous.

I am presenting you the most dramatic examples of how people get started on the guilt trip because I want to alert you to these possibilities. I am not suggesting that your own trip began in such a remarkable way. You may have never wished the person you care for would "drop dead." But before you completely dismiss this idea of your behavior being partially motivated by guilt, try to remember how you answered the question "What did I do to deserve this?" My hunch is that you came up with some answer.

Perhaps it was more like John's. John loved his fiancée and wanted to get married and settle down — but giving up other women was not going to be an easy chore. At his bachelor party, John had one last fling with an old high school sweetheart. After he returned from his honeymoon and moved into his new home, he was told by this old sweetheart that she was pregnant and needed money for an abortion. John borrowed money to pay for an abortion. .The girl went on her way, and John thought that would be the end of it. For him, though it was only the beginning. The following year, John's first child was born, a mentally retarded girl. In John's mind, this daughter represented the punishment for his past crime and he sacrificed his entire life — and eventually his marriage — trying to make this retarded daughter happy. He bought her fancy toys she couldn't use, bikes she couldn't ride, and lavish clothes she couldn't appreciate. He spent hour after hour reading to her stories she couldn't possibly understand.

Your crime or your punishment is not so obvious. When you asked yourself, "What did I do to deserve this?" you probably did not think of just one deed the way John did. Yes, you might have thought of that time you shoplifted as a teenager, or the time you let some guy take you all the way, or when you cheated on a final exam, but unlike John, it probably was not a single misdeed that made you feel that you were finally getting what you deserved. Rather, it was a general feeling about yourself that you were bad and should be punished. In a sense, you were feeling like the little girl who, when asked her name, said it was "Mary, don't! You're a bad girl!" I don't presume to know or why you had some basic feeling of being bad. It's not easy to uncover where that inherent sense of oneself comes from. What I do know is that many a ticket for the guilt trip has been purchased because the caregiver has a deep sense of being bad and makes inordinate sacrifices to try to overcome that feeling.

Am I already sounding too psychoanalytical, too mysterious? What is all this stuff about feeling bad or needing to be punished? All you know is that someone devoted his or her life to you and now you are in the position of paying that person back. We've heard all those types of explanations: "My father took care of me and supported me through school even though he could barely afford it"; "My mother saved for me and sacrificed her career for me"; "My husband bought me beautiful gifts and was always gentle with me." So what's so wrong about wanting to pay them back? Maybe nothing is wrong, but maybe everything. To be especially devoted to a person who was especially devoted to you is certainly not wrong. But ask yourself (honestly), would that person who loved you so dearly want you to "sacrifice your life" to the point that you feel burdened, oppressed, and limited in ability to work and play and love? You are in this fix because you are constantly thinking of and caring for that person who cared for you. You see, if you really believe that you deserved the love and sacrifice the other person gave you, then you will be able to respond to that person's needs in an appropriate manner. But if you suspect — somewhere down deep inside — that you were unworthy of the sacrifices the other person made for you, then you will overextend yourself in trying to pay him or her back.

By now, you may have gotten the mistaken idea that I think that guilt and responsibility for others is a bad thing and should be avoided. I believe no such thing. On the contrary, we all need a modicum of guilt to guide our behavior, to keep us in line, to help us get along with others. We need it to give us a little slap on the wrist when we screw up or to give us a pat on the back when we do something admirable. But a reasonable portion of guilt is not the reason the people become enmeshed in a Samaritan Syndrome. Their guilt is irrational and based on angry feelings towards the one for whom they care, or on bad feelings about themselves because of what they wished or what they did or what kind of person they think they are.

That is not to say that these feelings are not founded on a reality basis. Everyone at one time or another or has had evil thoughts.

Everyone has wished silently or out loud that something bad would happen to somebody else. Everyone, at some time or other, is rejected by a person he loves. The difference is that not everyone turns these thoughts or deeds into massive feelings of guilt, the kind of guilt that becomes crippling and further encumbers them and affects the disabled person as well. The journey that the Samaritan is on is not guided by reason but fueled by irrational guilt. If you think guilt was not a major factor in motivating you to buy a ticket on this trip, ask yourself what you imagine would happen if you stopped being saddled with the constant care of another. How would you feel if you turned this job over to another? Chances are, you'd feel more than just a little guilty. The punishment for not being the dutiful child, spouse, or parent would be far more drastic than that. You might believe you would drop dead or be affected by a dread disease or that you would end up in hell – if not a religious hell, then one you would make for yourself, your own private version.

Perhaps one of the important reasons for continuing this trip is the idea of what others might think of you. People who continually tell you what a saint you are or admire your patience and stamina might not think so highly of you if you stopped your caregiving role. The guilt you now feel would be multiplied by the guilt you know will be heaped upon you (or better yet, come from inside you) not only by the person you are serving, but also by all his loyal advocates.

Thus, I come to the crux of the matter. What motivates one to become a Samaritan? What made you take this trip to nowhere? The answer is largely guilt — guilt over imaginary deeds, guilt over real deeds, guilt over unspoken wishes, guilt over spoken anger. Because of this guilt, you made your choice to spend much of your lifetime devoted to an unfortunate person, caring for him at the expense of your own needs. The price is indeed high because guilt can be very expensive. There is no bargain basement guilt for you. Yours is more the boutique kind with boutique prices.

This analogy contains a thought to ponder. When you make a purchase, there is an option for you to take. There is a choice. The choice begins when you decide what store you go to shop and continues up to the point you pay for the purchase. Even then, you have a choice. You can exchange your purchase or give it away. This is true of the Samaritan Syndrome as well. Once you accept the fact that your motives for caring for someone are probably largely based on guilt (a shaky foundation at best), and that you have opted to do what you are doing for reasons that are not valid, you are ready to think about change. It's true that you have been in the same groove for so long, this thought may be so frightening that you have no clue as to how to make a different choice.

That's my job in subsequent chapters, to help you be aware of other alternatives and to help you realize that options are still open and that choices are still available. The very idea of changing your behavior no doubt makes you uncomfortable. However, I am not asking you to change anything yet – just keep asking yourself some honest questions.

Chapter 2

Buying the Ticket

The last chapter discussed ways that may have been a causal factor in your becoming a "Good Samaritan." It may seem as though I have lumped everyone in same group and see only stereotyped Samaritans. This is far from my intention. I am well aware of the differences in people, and though there may be a common thread running through the causation of this syndrome, people have their own idiosyncratic way of reacting. I do feel, however, the one basic ingredient is guilt.

In order to discuss the development of the syndrome and give you a chance to find yourself in this story, I have delineated five different types of caretakers — all stemming from the decision you made when you undertook this journey. These types describe how you might react to your situation as time passes and you feel stuck. Perhaps if you can identify with one of these scenarios, it might be easier to start thinking of the first step you might take to alleviate your "load" and see the sun and the stars again.

Caretaker Type 1

You view your partner's affliction as your fault. Although you recognize his problem is due to disease or age, you feel that you could have prevented the problem from developing or escalating if only you had been more thoughtful or a better person. You have assumed the largest part of the burden of your partnership. You seem to feel it is your responsibility to avoid all the pitfalls and control the course of the problem. You zealously guard your charge from all harm or outside interference. This, of course, causes you to neglect and suppress any other interests you might have or want to develop. Depending on your personality, you have found ways of adjusting to this lifestyle, stifling as it may be. In general, however, you feel you are atoning for past actions and must accept your limited life as inevitable and just.

You see the future as continuing in much the same way with little if any change. You cannot bear to think of life without your partner and will not plan ahead for that eventuality.

Caretaker Type 2

Your partnership is heavily weighted towards your side of the relationship. You recognize on one level that the problem belongs to your partner, but also feel it is your responsibility to ease the burden as much as possible. Because you do not fully accept the complete blame, there are times when you allow your partner to flounder by himself.

You convey to him that it's time he learned to help him a little. He may struggle with this notion for a while, and even make some headway. However, he soon realizes that life is much more comfortable for him when you are doing the greater part of the work. In his or her own peculiar style, he makes you aware that he is "sicker" than you thought and he is suffering unbelievable pain trying to please you. With a rush of "guilt", "love", "anxiety", or other emotional reaction, you scuttle to the rescue.

By reverting back to the onerous relationship, you drop any interest of your own that you may have been anticipating, probably with a mixture of resentment and relief. Each time you try to enable your partner to self-help and fail, you come more and more to the realization that there will be no release until death. With this thought, guilt raises its tyrannical head higher and you become more solicitous than you were before.

Caretaker Type 3

You have achieved what seems to be a reasonable partnership contract. The burden of the disorder is split in an equable way, with your partner accepting as much responsibility as he can for his needs and comfort. You, on the other hand, are there to lend support, both emotionally and physically. You recognize that his contribution to his physical and emotional care is limited by his disorder, perhaps severely so. In order to maintain your own equilibrium, you recognize that you will need help with the caregiving to cultivate and nurture your own interests and friends. You need these activities not only for your gratification, but also as a source of energy to enable you to be supportive. Therefore, you have created a reserve of auxiliary caregivers. To this end, you recruit family, friends, neighbors, and paid paraprofessionals who are ready to step in on a limited but steady basis. It is your job to leave as soon as the temporary caregiver arrives. An interesting fringe benefit of this arrangement is that your partner is stimulated by the variety of experiences with others.

Feeling good about yourself and your role allows you to enjoy his positive relationships with others and accept the resentment he may express when you go out on your own.

Caregiver Type 4

Although you have accepted a greater proportion of the distribution of labor, you firmly believe that the problem is not yours but a result of the disorder and your partner's way of coping with it. You may even believe in your heart, perhaps irrationally, that somehow he caused it to happen and you are the victim of his actions. You don't know why or even remember how you became the only one to shoulder the burden. There are other family members, but they are deaf and blind when it comes to helping out or even taking over. Although you feel so resentful, you put on a contented face for the rest of the world. You show enthusiasm that you don't feel, devotion to your partner that is only partially true, and have even learned to joke about the situation. No one understands or even pretends to understand the truth of the matter.

Annie was the youngest of five children. Bill was next to the youngest and they were very close. The older siblings married and the parents went to a retirement village. Annie and Bill each had his own apartments but kept in touch. Bill was an active man and loved doing recreational sports that bordered on the dangerous side. On one rafting trip, an unexpected storm came up and the raft capsized. He couldn't move his legs and spent several hours floating in the cold water until he was rescued. His injuries were severe and both his legs were amputated. The family rallied around, but once he was ready to leave rehab, everyone needed to return home, and Anne said that she would move in with him for a while. The "while" became permanent despite her requests for relief. Anne knew Bill could do more for himself because he had done so in rehab. However, he was so angry and despondent that Anne found it easier to do all, then to endure Bill's surly attitude. Her dreams of an independent life remained just a dream.

Like Anne, you do ask him sporadically to take responsibility on a limited basis. Even if he does, you can't help seeing how hard he struggles. Your feelings of being aggrieved by the situation encourage you to "take over." This becomes a dance you actively participate in – urging him to do more, then sabotaging his attempt. He retaliates by finding ways to manipulate you so that you become his slave (willingly or unwillingly).

You both become enmeshed in this scenario. Your life has been taken over. You don't know why or even remember how you became the only one to shoulder the burden. The other family members still maintain they cannot have a more active role in the caregiving. Although you feel resentful, you put on a contented face for the rest of the world. You show enthusiasm that you don't feel, devotion to your partner that is only partially true, and have even learned to joke about the situation. No one understands or even pretends to understand the truth of the matter.

You are denied any chance of achieving your goals, even though at this point you have forgotten what you dreamed of doing. As time goes on, you realize that there will never be any relief and you will spend your entire life bound to this task.

Caregiver Type 5

You are convinced that the situation was his entire fault. Rational or irrational, you maintain in your thoughts all the reasons why your partner is to blame. "He didn't watch his"; "He or could control his psychosis if he wanted to"; "He may be retarded, but if he would only pay attention, he would be more independent"; "He wouldn't be so crippled if he would try harder to use his limbs"; "He may be old and forgetful, but he doesn't have to be so needy" and whatever else you can think of that would lessen your load. Because of your beliefs, you feel are the victim, not your partner. How did you get into this situation in the first place? Why should you be punished for someone else's woes? If you were free, you could do so much with your life. You are not sure what you would do, but certainly anything but this. These feelings make you extremely angry. You lose your temper with your partner, and that only makes things worse. He tries to please you but is so scared you will leave him that he screws up. The circle goes round and round and the rut you are in gets deeper and deeper. You know you are doomed for the rest of your life.

As an example, let's look at Laura's situation. Laura was an executive secretary at a large corporation. She and Richard were married when they were both in their late twenties. Married life was great and they were thinking about having children. Then Richard discovered he had diabetes. The doctors prescribed a regimen of diet and exercise that would help him control the condition. He was warned about the possible complications that could occur if the diabetes became out of control. Richard was scared, and for a week or so, heeded the doctor's advice. Then he began to "cheat" a little on the diet and soon was eating all the forbidden foods. Laura's arguments and tears had no effect. He announced he was tired of this stupid diet; he was okay now and could live his life his way. His sugar went out of control and all the complications he had been warned about began to surface. He finally reached the point when he could no longer work, and indeed could do little of anything. Laura tried working part-time but could not handle all the emergency calls. She appealed to his mother to help her out. His mother refused. She "would love to help" but she "had a very busy life" and besides, Laura was his wife and he was her responsibility. Laura finally gave up her job, one she really loved, to stay home and take care of him. Although she did not say anything to him, she resented him for not following instructions and thus landing both of them in an impossible situation. Having children was out of the question, and all Laura could see ahead was a life of drudgery. She resented giving up her career, but they were married and that was that.

These five descriptions represent roughly the relationship between caretaker and caregiver. As with all typecasting, you probably do not fit exactly in any one of them. You may be somewhere in between or you might say they are all off the wall and do not describe you! However, before you close the book and toss it away, have a good long look at yourself. I'm sure you will find one type that sort of describes you. You may have to do some painful introspection to arrive at this conclusion, but remember how long it took to get where you are. The reason it is so important to identify with one of these scenarios is to give you a baseline to work from.

Though Type 3 seems to be the best compromise, arriving at that point from where you are could be a very short journey or a long and difficult one with many detours. You must remember that less is more and that changing your situation will be arduous and slow.

Looking at yourself may be painful. Keep in mind you can't really change your partner's behavior. What you can do is change the way you act and react to him, and that in turn should slowly change his attitude and behavior. The starting place is you, how you are now and where you would like to be. The journey will be filled with pitfalls and disappointments, but hopefully this book will serve as a guide to your destination. Unlike a travel guide, I can't exactly map the route, but I can suggest the major highways, the scenic routes, and alert you to the detours.

Chapter 3

Sin of Kin

When trouble strikes someone near and dear to you, you feel shocked, alone, and helpless. You want someone to share this with you. You want some one to comfort you, to support you, and make you feel that things will somehow work out. Usually you expect family to serve this role. After all, family is people you've known all your life, people who love you and whom you love and trust to help you. Usually, family does rise to the occasion during the acute stage of illness or the beginning of your knowledge of the scope of disability. However, when the immediate crisis is over, everyone returns to his "normal life," happy with the knowledge that you will be responsible for the ongoing care, and they can rely on you to do the job.

Of course, you did agree to be the caregiver. Of course, you did expect that the family would help and support you. The help you need may be actual hands-on labor such as "Help me move my belongings to accommodate the new partner"; "Help me bathe him"; "Help me with the shopping"; or "Help me with the expenses." Inwardly, what you are craving more than the actual help is moral support. You need assurance that things will work out.

And in the beginning of this saga, family is there for you. They know the pains both of you are experiencing, and since they are not cold-hearted or uncaring, they try to pitch in. The hands-on aid, however, dwindles and you get promises to help, promises that more often than not are broken. The shock and the novelty have worn off and people start to call instead of coming over. Then the calls become more infrequent until they practically stop. Why does this happen? One reason is the "there but for the grace of God go I" syndrome. Then too, you are not as much fun as you used to be or even as interesting. You are so wrapped up in the caring process that you have no time to do anything else, certainly go anywhere else, or even keep up with world outside of your sphere. You become more and more isolated until your relationship is with your partner alone and your concerns are centered on his well-being.

The retreat of family support is slow and insidious. The problem is a long-term one. It won't get better or go away. It is when friends and family realize this reality, that they openly or tacitly back away and delegate the care to you. They appoint you chief custodian, provider, nurse, caregiver, or whatever title you choose to call yourself. They return to their own lives. It doesn't matter if they continue to live in the same house or are 3,000 miles away. The important issue is that they reviewed the situation, and decided that they did not want the glory of being chief cook and bottle washer. The responsibility is delegated to you. They have abdicated and given you the throne.

This was Bea's experience. Bea lived near her mother. She had a successful career as a teacher and a few friends with whom she socialized. She tried faithfully to have a weekend date to lunch with her mother. During one of these lunches, her mother suddenly fell off the chair. She was rushed to the hospital and it was soon apparent she had had a massive stroke. Bea's two sisters and her brother rushed to their mother's side. One lived across country, the others fairly close by. As Mother went from hospital to rehab, it became apparent that she could not live alone without a caregiver. At first, the siblings agreed to chip in to pay a companion, but this idea passed as soon as they discovered how much home care costs. Bea reluctantly consented to move in temporarily, until they all could come up with a solution. They did, and the solution was that Bea should stay for a while longer. She took a leave of absence but eventually realized she would have to resign. Taking care of her mother was an arduous job. Bea begged her siblings for some actual help. No one even had time to visit for more than a few hours. They were usually on their way somewhere and did not have time to do any chores. However, they were profuse in their praise of how wonderful it was of Bea to take care of Mom. When the idea of sharing the cost of a helper was again proposed, all the siblings brought up the dreadful expenses they incurred with the big house and private schools. Much as they would like to chip in, Bea had to realize no one could help financially. Ironically, June —who lived the farthest — did leave her family every January to spend two weeks with her mother and sister. June was freaked out by the actual chores, but at least she lent moral support. Of course, she found fault with Bea's routine, and during the rest of the year gave advice based on "I noticed when I stayed with you that there is a better way to do that." Bea kept her resentment to herself, fearful that even the yearly visits would stop. The years slipped by and Bea was "the wonderful daughter who sacrificed for Mom."

Family members can find all kind of excuses to abdicate the responsibility. But if the truth is to be known, they want to remain the power behind the throne. The day-by-day care and endless chores are all yours, but someone else wants to be the prime minister or secretary of state, go to all the meetings, address the Congress, meet with all the other heads of state, and advise you of their decisions. Others want to be members of Congress, debate the issues and pass the laws. Others want to judge, hear the case and decide if the laws are justified or if the decisions of the lower court should be reversed. However, you are allowed to be the executive, deprived of all the executive powers. The secretary of state, the Congress, and the judges, (from a comfortable distance) real or imagined, tell you how to care for your charge.

This analogy may sound somewhat silly and far-fetched. The metaphors are puffed up, but this overstatement points out how pompous and righteous other family members can be. It also illustrates that they regard you as inferior to them and not nearly as wise. The worst part is that they have no idea how hurtful this attitude is to you.

Katie's mom was distraught when her husband died. She was the consummate example of the wife of the 1930s. She managed the household, took care of the kids, and her husband gave her a weekly allowance for food. She never had to pay a bill or cope with a checking account. When her husband died, she literally did not know how to take care of herself or was she about to learn. The three daughters decided she had to live with one of them. Susan said she would gladly take Mom, but she was so busy with their new business that she would never be home for her. Alice said she also would be happy to take Mom, but now was a bad time. The house was small and already overcrowded with her four kids. When they bought a bigger house, it would be easier for her to take Mom. That left Kate. Kate was between part-time jobs then, and the children were in college or about to go, so she agreed to have Mom come live with her family for now. But she made it clear that at some point, the other sisters would arrange for Mom to live with them. Of course, once Mom was ensconced in Katie's house, the moon would turn green before anything changed. At first, it was okay. Mom was desolate and demanded constant attention, but Kate thought eventually Mom would try to help. She was a good cook, but she never used and was slightly afraid of the electric stove. No matter how often Kate tried to teach her how the stove worked, she would refuse to learn. However, she constantly found fault with Katie's cooking.

And so it went, and as the years slipped by, contending with her became more and more difficult, especially after her vision and hearing began to fail. Katie's complaints to her sisters did not fall on deaf ears. On the contrary, Susan's litany was "If you only were more patient with her, she wouldn't be so difficult. You were always stubborn and unreasonable. Grow up and let her have her way once in a while."

Alice maintained, "You are a patsy. You were always easy to take advantage of. You just lie down and let everyone walk right over you. Mom always did and Alan (Katie's husband) treats you like a dishrag... Just lay down the law!" These opinions were always followed by, "She doesn't act that way when I'm around" (which, by the way was very seldom). Her mom became a full-time job. Katie's children had their own lives now and her husband hardly ever came home before midnight and left as soon as he got up. Katie was stuck, and all she ever got from everyone was criticism.

Like Katie's sisters, your relatives probably advise you of excellent, well-thought-out suggestions. They may berate you or bemoan the idiotic way you manage. If only they "could," they "would do a much better job." However, after reciting all the important things they have to do, they concede, with a sigh (of relief?) that since you are the designated one, you will continue to muddle through your daily routine. It's true; you don't have much of a life, but that's your own fault. You just refuse to follow sensible advice. Their suggestions would, in their opinion, make life much easier for the suffering person. Although at this point it's hard to distinguish whom that one might be – you or your partner.

What makes all this more difficult is the effect the absent prime minister seems to have on your partner. The longer a loved one stays away, the more stature he attains. Aunt Sadie, who shows up one day a year to visit her "poor afflicted sister," is greeted with hugs and kisses and tears of joy. Brother John, who flies in twice a year for five minutes, is rewarded with a glowing smile. Those drop-ins or drop-outs — depending on your point of view — seem to be the favored relations, while you, the faithful, the drudge, the always-there-when-I-need-you person, are never right, seldom complimented, and often the object of abuse.

Greta, unlike Katie and Bea, willingly offered to take Mom. She was the youngest of four, and as a child had been the butt of her siblings' jokes. She was good in school (which caused some jealousy) but awkward and clumsy when she tried to ride a bike or play tennis. She strove to please Mom by running errands and helping around the house while the others were succeeding at sports and having dates. When Mom began to fail, Greta took her to live with her family. Mom was tough and obstinate, but Greta suffered in silence, still trying to gain points. Mom rarely had a good word to say about her, but talked constantly about the success of her other children and how wonderful their kids were (even if she rarely saw them). When Mom had to be hospitalized, Greta spent all day at her bedside, prepared her favorite food and endured her complaints. Mom anticipated her other children's visits, telling the nurses how sweet it was for them to find the time to visit her, and she absolutely beamed when they came. Greta learned not to be sarcastic, because Mom would defend them and tell her she shouldn't be so jealous.

Absence, in this case, does not really make the heart grow fonder. What it does is allow both parties to distance themselves from each other. For your partner, distance enhances the kind and caring traits that he remembers and dulls the characteristics that are annoying and grate on his nerves. As far as the faraway person is concerned, temper tantrums aren't so bad when you aren't subjected to them on a regular basis. Drunken sprees seem less threatening when you are not faced with the aftermath of violence or sickness. Absent-mindedness or the forgetfulness due to organic deterioration is not as horrendous when you don't have to make sure that the gas jets are turned off or the lighted cigarette was not dropped and smoldering in the bed or chair.

To add insult to injury, the absentee's propensity to forget birthdays or other important occasions is excused when they call with apologies and explain how busy they are. Their tendency to be bossy or dominating is tolerable from a distance. Chances are that when they do appear on the scene, they are perky, unperturbed, and delighted to finally be here, especially since "I can't stay too long." These visitors were always treated with pleasantness and good cheer because your partner is afraid of losing them altogether. He knows from experience that the absent relative can and does stay away for extended periods of time. Therefore, he thinks "if I am not nice to him, he may stay away longer, or perhaps never come back." The anger one may feel because the absentee doesn't come more often is not expressed. Instead, rationalizations for the absence must be expressed. Rather than feel the absentee stay away because he doesn't care, your partner would rather feel "he stays away because he has so many other demands on his time and money. I must enjoy him while he is here, to insure that he will come back." This attitude is not designed to make you feel appreciated.

For example, Alice spent three years caring for her mother-in-law, who was dying a slow and painful death. The mother-in-law's daughter, who lived fifty miles away, would call and bemoan the fact that she just couldn't bring herself to visit Mom more often. "You don't understand how hard it is for me to watch her suffer." The implication is that you have no feeling and can callously watch the suffering. Mom, on the other hand, when daughter does call, will "understand how hard it is to drive so far." After the phone call, Mom will spend three days talking about her "wonderful Zelda." As the caring daughter-in-law, you may spend many an hour fantasizing how you would like to torture Zelda. The favorite fantasy that evolves is not to murder her in numerous ingenious ways, but to lock her in the room with Mom and not let her out for two weeks.

This is rather a healthy fantasy for the caregiver whose feelings were being trod upon and whose efforts were being ignored. Perhaps it was a little easier for her to endure the insults, knowing that Mom's life expectancy was severely limited by her illness. Knowing that she might have to endure many more years of "wonderful Zelda" will have created much more entrenched resentment and bitterness.

Distant relatives and even not-so-distant relatives have discovered another ploy to make you continue in your role. It's the "aren't-you-wonderful-to-be-so-devoted-to-dear-whomever." They encourage you and work hard at being a great cheering squad. If you manage to squeak out a complaint or suggest that the role is getting to you and you don't know how long you can continue, the panicked relatives rush to assure you that you enjoy what you are doing. "You're just feeling a little blue right now. You know that so-and-so adores you. Get some more rest and you'll feel better soon."

The corollary to this approach is that "I'm not as wonderful as you. I haven't the patience you have, and you are doing such a great job." Translation: "If you stop doing this, then I might have to get involved." Thus, when you show signs of weakening, you can rest assured that you will be cajoled into continuing.

The concomitant approach is the belief that you are the natural one for this role. She is your wife or your daughter or your mother. Or he is your husband, your son, or your father. This becomes a bit tricky when your wife happens to be the other person's mother, but it makes sense if you are the other person. Sounds a little confusing? Let's try to make it a little clearer.

Mr. Jones, at age fifty-five, has a stroke and is left severely impaired. Mrs. Jones quits her job and stays home to take care of her husband. The three children feel terrible about poor Dad, but think it is wonderful (and fortuitous) that he has Mom to take care of him. Now, if Mom is to fade out of the picture (probably due to overwork and stress) one of the children will take over or make other arrangements. But, as long as Mom is around, she is the natural custodian and the children feel no obligation to help out, except in extraordinary circumstances, for a brief time. This might be because Mom succumbs to pneumonia or some other temporary, perhaps life-threatening condition. The message that Mom receives and accepts is that this is now her job and hers alone. Like you, she realizes that the caregiver has tenure and cannot be fired. Indeed there is a clause in the "contract" that says you can never resign!

Another device kinfolk use to convince themselves (and you if possible) is that it is right for you to take sole care of your afflicted relative is because you will profit in the long run. When dear old Aunt Sarah finally passes on, you will inherit all her worldly possessions. These may range from a large estate to her rather comfortable home to her sterling service for twenty-four, or perhaps just her Wedgwood bowl. Whatever possessions are left will probably be up for grabs when the time comes, but in the meantime, that's a useful rationalization for the rest of the family. This may be your motive, but it's doubtful that it is the sole incentive in light of what I have already discussed. In most instances, whatever you receive will be rather small payment for many years of labor. Figured on an hourly basis, it may come out to well under minimum wage. For the rest of the family, however, as long as you are taking care of the unfortunate relative, the estate becomes larger and larger, the house worth a fortune, and the Wedgwood bowl a priceless antique. Of course, by the time you claim your prize, you too may be a worn-out antique. It is also possible that when the time comes, the family will assert their rights and squabble after the "fortune."

Helen and Harry were down on their luck and went to stay with Mom in her house. Harry had time on his hands so began to repair and renovate the house. All this was fine until Mom became eighty-five years old and broke her hip. She never fully recovered and was unable to walk. Since she was on Medicaid, the city paid for the home aide. As Mom neared ninety-five and real estate values increased, the other children began to worry that Helen and Harry might claim the house when she died. A search for a will was fruitless, and no one could persuade Mom to make one. The squabbles became so heated that Helen and Harry were not on speaking terms with the other children. When Mom succumbed, the others went to a lawyer. Much to their chagrin, the law stated that the house had to be sold to satisfy the Medicaid bills (by this time phenomenal). However, this process was delayed as long as the resident children lived in the house. The truth was that Helen and Harry may not have taken actual personal care of Mom, but they had lived there for fifteen years and monitored her welfare. Was that fair? You decide.

Let us move on to the insurmountable rationale – the geographical cop-out. With a deep sigh, kinfolk say, "I would love to help you out if only I lived closer, but a thousand miles is so far away. I'm lucky if I can get there once a year." The actual mileage doesn't really matter, since the geographical cop-out can encompass any distance that is further than next door. The distance reflects an attitude adopted by others to defend themselves against their own feelings of kinship obligation. As a wise old grandmother I know whose English is rather colorful and expressive, says, "Where there's a want-to, there's a can." Distance can be shortened or lengthened depending upon what one is motivated to do. Those who cling to the geographical excuse are convinced it is valid, even if you are not.

Finally, the *piece de resistance,* the non-arguable excuse is what we call the "you-think-you-have-problems!" argument. Those who use this ploy know that the best defense is an offense. When you venture to complain about your plight, you don't get sympathy. Instead you hear about how difficult life is for sister Joan. "I'm being run ragged trying to keep this big house clean with only part-time help. Jim doesn't get home till eight, so by the time we eat dinner and get the dishes done, we've missed all the good TV movies and I'm so exhausted, I must to go to bed in order to face the next day. I just don't know how I'm going to be ready to go to Europe in four weeks with all I have to do – shopping and packing and making arrangements for the dog." Somehow, you get the feeling that you would be more than willing to trade your problems for hers, but can't get a word in edgewise. Besides, she's much better at one-upmanship than you are, so you decide it's a losing battle to challenge her.

Perhaps your family doesn't seem to fit in any of these categories. However, if you think about it, you'll be sure to discover that whatever pretext they use, the excuses are designed to achieve one major purpose: to convince you that caring for someone else is exactly what you ought to be doing. It relieves everyone else of the responsibility and allows them to go on with their own lives, convinced that your partner is receiving the best of all possible care. They are right about that – indeed he is.

The reason why these various rationalizations succeed will be discussed in the next chapter, which has to do with you and your needs.

Chapter 4

Use of Abuse

Most of us learn at a very early age that all deeds have consequences. If our parents were completely consistent and we lived in an ideal world, all good deeds would have good consequences and all bad acts would have bad consequences. Since parents are rarely perfect, and other imperfect people influence us as well, life's experiences hardly ever fall into black-and-white categories. Good deeds may go unnoticed and bad deeds may be rewarded. It's possible to help your little brother clean up his toys and not even get a thank you, or to cheat on a test and get an A. Things we enjoy may be considered taboo and things we hate get rave notices. For example, your mother may not let you watch the violent shows you think are terrific, but be thrilled when you eat up all your spinach. This being the case, we grow up with confused notions of good and bad. Often, what we enjoy is deemed bad by our instilled notions, and good defined by disappointing and duty-bound chores.

Jimmy discovered finger paints at school and was fascinated by the patterns he made. Every day, he asked the teacher if he could finger-paint. However, when he brought his pictures to his mom, she said they were ugly and screamed that the paint ruined his clothes... Thus, he learned that an activity he loved was "bad." He also learned that "dirty" was bad. As a grown-up, he was overly concerned with cleanliness. His apartment sparkled from his constant scrubbing and polishing. After marriage, he continued to do most of the cleaning because "he was better at it than she was."

When grown, we may do what is "good for us," but privately hunger to satisfy the needs that we learned are bad for us. Our need to satisfy those secret and "bad" needs is strong, though we are usually unconscious of the reason. We all feed our inner hunger in our own unique way, and for the most part are unaware of the process.

Overeating is one method of sating inner needs. Stan snacked all the time. He stuffed himself with junk food, completely ignoring the nagging of his wife and the advice of his doctor. When diagnosed with diabetes, the nagging and admonitions became stronger and constant. Nevertheless, he continued to satisfy his craving for sweets, often on the sly to avoid the criticism. He was completely unaware that eating was a way of satisfying his frustrated hidden needs. As a little boy, his mother always had chocolate cake and milk waiting for him when he came home from school. Whenever he cried or complained of an injustice, Mother gave him something to eat. "Eat, son. You'll feel better" was her theme song. He gained so much weight that the boys in school made fun of him. So he ate to feel better. He matured, but his need to be comforted by food did not. Since he never connected eating with these early satisfactions, he continued to maintain that he ate sweets because needed the enhanced energy level to function.

Knowing that our significant adults will not condone needs that are "bad" or "sinful" or "unworthy," we learn at an early age to keep the satisfaction of those needs under wraps or disguised. Many a forbidden comic book is hidden and read inside the geography book. Children, teenagers, and adults do prohibited, wicked things and hope nobody finds out. Since we receive and absorb these very mixed messages while growing up, it is understandable that we think that we are doing "good" for very altruistic reasons. In truth, we may be doing good to satisfy an inner need that is quite the opposite. All behavior has meaning, but the meaning is often muddled and unclear.

Take Aaron, for example. Aaron's mother was a hypercritical person. Nobody could meet her standards of an excellent job. Indeed, even a well-done job was never quite right. Aaron's father was rarely home (not hard to imagine why) and Aaron "ineptly" did all the chores. In school, he usually achieved a B average, which of course was not an A. As Aaron grew to adulthood, he no longer tried to please his dissatisfied mother. However, at work, he always volunteered for any task, pleasant or not.

He thought he did this to advance his status at the firm (and indeed it did) but he never considered that he still longed to satisfy his mother. Incidentally, she thought his progress was too slow!

Samantha offered to be the caregiver when older sister Mandy was confined to a wheelchair. Everyone admired her unselfishness and devotion to her sister. She said she was glad she could help, and basked in the accolades. It never dawned on her that her "doing good" assuaged the guilt she had felt for a long time. As a young teenager, she was very jealous of her sister's popularity. Whenever she could, she would tell Mandy's boyfriends mean things about her sister. Most of these stories were lies, but she succeeded in sabotaging Mandy's social life. Mandy never understood why so many of the boys dropped her, and Samantha was not about to tell. Now they were middle-aged women and Samantha had long ago blocked all of this from her memory. Devoting her energies to Mandy's plight was not as altruistic as even she thought. In reality, she was meeting her hidden need to atone.

We explore in this chapter, motives that are not apparent on the surface. It is safe to say, these motives may also not be apparent to ourselves. It will be a difficult to think about because it is troubling to look at ourselves with an unprejudiced, dispassionate view. However, in order to effect change, you must know what you want to change and why you want to change it. You also need to understand what is keeping you from making that change. What are you getting from the present situation? How is that satisfying your needs? It is a revolutionary thought that even though you feel you are trapped, even though you are tired of constantly doing for someone else, even though you feel that your desires are unfulfilled, in some way, you are receiving strokes that make you feel good. Somehow, this situation supports a lifestyle that internally satisfies you.

This does not imply that victims enjoy being victimized, but a bad situation may persist because your early life plays some part in accepting and continuing the despised role. Inner needs are being met, needs that you have kept hidden for a long time. You will have to dig deep to recognize them, and may find yourself wincing all the way.

How do you start? The first step is scrutinizing your role in the family when you were a youngster. Don't reject this approach because it sounds too analytical. We do not grow up in a vacuum, nor do we grow up in an ideal setting. Our childhood roles fashion us into the person we are today, both the person we show to the world and believe we are, and the person we have buried inside.

Suppose for a minute you were like Jody. She was the oldest in the family and was appointed Mother's helper. From the time she learned to tie her own shoes, she was responsible for overseeing her younger siblings while they were getting dressed. Her responsibilities grew as the family grew, and her duties made her feel very grown-up. Sometimes she would rather be doing her own age-related activities, but she stifled those thoughts. She relished the importance of her role and her domination over the other kids. Is it plausible to think that role Jody played in the family affected her business and personal life when she was grown? Of course, she remembered taking care of the kids. She just could not acknowledge the feelings she stifled. She didn't recognize the resentment she felt toward her mother. She denied the times she hated her siblings and wished they would all suddenly disappear. When overwhelmed by her responsibilities, she was more demanding of the younger kids. However, all of these feelings were stirred up when she assumed a caregiving role. Her only way of defending against them came from years of practice. She refused all help and was trapped in her situation.

I assume for our purposes that you did not grow up in an overtly dysfunctional family, the kind of dysfunctional families depicted on TV and in movies. These portrayals probably do not describe your family of origin. Dysfunctional families tend to make interesting stories. There are good guys and bad guys. They are inconsistent in behavior and interaction. Sometimes one member is dominating or fearful and the others meek or avoidant. Sometimes greed and mayhem are usual atmospheres. Sometimes delinquency is rampant. These dysfunctional ways of interaction with each other results in distorted character development and an uncontrollable family life. This may be your background, but most of us of us grew up in a family that works reasonably well. No one is overtly delinquent or unmanageable, although each may have foibles that grate on one's nerves. A family like Jody's may not have given her a fair shake, but the family survived very well.

Whether you grew up as an only child or with many siblings, each one in your family had an influence on you. Were your parents so busy that they had little time for you? Did your older brother bully you? Did your family tease you a lot? Was your older sister beautiful with perfect features? Was there a child that you considered the favorite one? Were you known as the "brain in the family" or the "dummy"? Were your ideas listened to or laughed at? Were you lonely much of the time? Did you have few friends, or were you a social butterfly?

Not only should you attempt to answer these questions (and some others you think of that I didn't pose) but also try to think about the lasting effects. Make no mistake about it. Everyone else, including you, may have forgotten these everyday events, but how you felt at that time has a lasting effect on your overt and covert behavior. Admonitions such as "don't be a baby"; "there's nothing to cry about"; "you shouldn't let that frighten you"; "that's not important"; "I have no time no time listen to you whine"; "go away and leave me alone"; and "you'll be the death of me" if said often enough, will make you feel rejected, lonely, or unimportant. You and you alone must dig down and realize how events in your family or school life made you feel inside.

This is not an easy task. Since most of us want to make a "good" impression, it makes sense to all hide unwanted feelings from others as well as ourselves. That hidden feeling of rejection may make you eager to please today. Feeling squashed then may be why you feel like a dishrag now. Feeling inadequate then may make do things you really don't want to do in order to please. I could go on and on, but I think you get the idea now. It's not just the things we remember that make us what we are today, the feelings we repressed and the events we pushed away may have a big influence on how we live our lives now.

Ginny takes meticulous care of her ailing mother and reels in horror at the thought of getting help. She does not realize that her almost fanatical need to be responsible stems from early years. She was an only child, born after fifteen years of marriage. Her parents had given up hope of ever conceiving a baby and considered her their "miracle child." Her mother's insecurity made her a constant worrier. Although she tried to not reveal her fears to her child, her fears of something terrible happening to Ginny almost exuded from her pores. She was an extremely intelligent woman, but so paralyzed by her anxiety that whenever Ginny was hurt, she would call her husband at work to ask him what to do. Ginny internalized the idea that dangers always lurked in the world, and that one must always be alert. At the same time, she resented her mother's "over concern." It cast a pall on her activities with other kids and intensified her own childhood fears. When her mother became bedridden, Ginny's compulsive care stemmed from her childhood overprotection and resentment of being so constrained.

Now that you have some understanding of underlying motives and hopefully have uncovered some of your own hidden needs, we will look at how the caregiver role may be fueled by these needs. One aspect of your present situation is that you are never alone. The other person in your life may not be the best companion in the world and far from ideal, but he is company. He will not leave you, because he needs to be cared for. Do you stay because you are the one person in the entire world who can care for him? Think about it. How much do you fear being alone and having no one in your life?

You are also essential to you partner's functioning, in fact, as far as he is concerned, the most important person in his life. You are always aware of the unpleasant aspects of caring for him. For example, a severely retarded adult is not intellectually stimulating. He probably needs help with toileting and hygiene, and must be constantly supervised. However, he can also be affectionate and playful, a child forever. He is very needy and you are his whole world. As a matter of fact, no matter what the handicapping condition may be, dependency is the general characteristic common to all. The person may not like to be helpless, and object voraciously. That, however, is not the issue. The issue is that you will always have someone who needs you. Do you get satisfaction from knowing someone would be lost without you?

Thus, having a companion and being needed by that person can give you a sense of well-being underneath the anger and resentment. The relationship that grows between you and the problem-laden person is nourished by his dependency despite the arguments and harsh words. You are both playing an essential role and you both profit from it. The term "caretaker" is often used as the designation of the healthy person. We avoid using this term, for as you give thought to the situation and scrutinize it, the relationship between the two individuals involved may make you question just who the caretaker is. The one who does all the work, or the one receiving the benefits of the work? Substituting *caregiver* for one and *care recipient* for the other seems to be more accurate. The principles espoused in this chapter beg the question of who gives and who receives. This relationship, as in any other (good or bad), results in both receiving something from it, be it pleasant or disagreeable.

Take, for example, the following situation. A couple has been married for fifty years. He is forgetful with organic problems, but spry and agile. She is intellectually sound and alert, but her mobility is impaired. She handles the finances; he cleans the house. She is his head, and he serves as her legs. When he is confused, he attacks her and she retaliates with her cane. They are both bruised, and the frustration and anger are extremely visible. However, when you spend time with them, you are struck by their concern for each other. It becomes very obvious that their overriding fear is that one will die and leave the other alone. Weird? Maybe. But it works for them. Abusive? Yes. But each gets something out of it and both will be devastated without the other. The boundary dividing caregiver from care recipient is blurred, and in this case, it is impossible to distinguish one from the other.

This case is well-defined and clear-cut. Yours may not be quite as simple. However, it is very apparent that one is stalwart and the other is not. The fact remains that if one of you goes, the other is left alone. Your partner, out of necessity, will have to be attended either by another person or an institution. If he goes first, however, you will be totally alone. How frightening is that for you? Chances are, the thought of no longer being a slave is a relief; the loneliness is difficult to conceive. Though consciously, you may be aware of the inevitable loneliness, unconsciously you may be terrified.

The discussion about the "use of abuse" means exploring in depth the reasons why you are "stuck." What is going on that encourages you to stay, other than a sense of duty? Well, for one thing, friends and relatives play a role in this complicated relationship. Since none of them wish to take over your role, they work hard to keep you ensconced in that position. Even though they criticize and advise, the overwhelming message is "Thank heavens you are made of the stuff to take care of mom/sister/father/child/whoever, because I might have to take over if you quit." You may recognize that you are getting a "snow job," but it is gratifying to hear you are so patient, saintly, kindhearted, gentle, giving, devoted, and worthy of a gold throne in heaven. Others admire you (from a safe distance) and honor you (from afar). Your partner also feeds this admiration. He realizes when you are reaching the end of your rope and feels threatened by the thought you might leave. That is when he clings to you and conveys how important you are to him (as indeed you are!) and how much he needs you (which indeed he does). This adoration may be spotty, but when you feel this adulation, it is hard to dismiss the effect. It softens the many hours of abuse and drudgery.

Strange as it may sound, these are some of the more obvious rewards of your plight. There are other more subtle incentives to stay within the confines of your relationship rather than venture forward. The most apparent disadvantage of this situation is being boxed in and unable to go out. How does this work for you? Your emphatic response is probably "Not at all." Let's think about it. Turn the question from "What do I miss by not being free to go out?" to "What hassles do I avoid by being locked in?" For one thing, enmeshed in your present association means you do not have to get involved in any other liaison. Other liaisons are risky, and by entering into one, you risk being rejected, risk being hurt, and most importantly, risk being vulnerable to defeat. What you are doing now, you know you do well. What lies outside may be quite different and possibly involve defeat. Chances are, you have been locked in so long that the thought of what's outside is scary. You may think about being free, dream about it, and fervently wish for it. Could you really cope with the outside world after being confined for so long? Could you deal with a more equitable relationship after being comfortably, if not happily, enmeshed with your present companion?

Paul dreamed of having an "important position." His job as a Realtor was interesting; he was good at it and enjoyed the financial rewards. Still, he wanted to experience more prestige and pizzazz. He decided that being in politics might be exciting. He joined a political club and eventually was asked to run for mayor of his rather small town. He was flattered and anxious to win. His enthusiasm was dampened when he had to make his first campaign speech. He was overwhelmed. For the first time, he thought about the duties and responsibilities of the job. He was used to people liking him, and worried that this might not be the case if elected. He thought of the decisions he would have to make, and how his neighbors might react to them. In effect, he was so scared of real and imagined ramifications that he withdrew his candidacy before the campaign even got started.

Similarly, what do you fear might happen if you gave up your present responsibilities? How would you cope with making new friends? Would you find new interests? Could you handle new and different situations? Could you face failing or finding out you have limitations? These are hard questions to answer honestly. Is what you are doing, as difficult as it is, easier to deal with than the unknown? How frightening are the obstacles you would have to tackle? Let's move on to anther issue.

We all know the story of Peter Pan, the little boy who never wanted to grow up and "wear a suit and tie and go to work every day." He created a haven where he could be a boy forever and avoid the responsibilities of manhood. The principle applies to girls as well, girls who do not want to grow up and do womanly things. For example, let's talk about Wendy, the little girl who happily flew away with Peter Pan. Wendy presents a different set of dynamics. Wendy is a sweet adolescent girl who is captivated by the charm and romance of the "forever" boy. She is intrigued by his promises of a carefree, exciting life in Never-Never Land. All she would have to do is mother the "lost boys." Peter paints a picture of a place where one never grows old – a land where there's naught but fun and adventure — a land where one may play forever. So Wendy decides to give up the world where she knows she will have to grow up, for a land of fantasy. She spreads her wings and off they go. Peter and her brothers indeed have a "funderful" time. But what is Wendy doing when she is not having fun? She is keeping house for the Peter and her brothers, cooking meals, mending clothes, and becoming an overworked surrogate mother. She never stops worrying about the welfare of her charges. Her responsibilities grow, and soon she has all the "lost boys" under her wing as well as Peter and her brothers. The Never-Never Land she dreamed about becomes an unpleasant reality. Finally, Wendy leaves and returns to her parents, saddened but relieved. She accepts the fact that she must grow up and undertake the responsibilities of marriage and children in a real world. (Changing times may mean a career in a demanding job, with or without marriage). The Wendy Syndrome can be defined as a flight from the real world to a make-believe world of pleasure. However, unlike the Peter Pan's Never-Grow-Up Land, Wendy's pretend world turned out to be an encapsulated segment of the world she thought she escaped. In her Never-Never Land, she retained the worries, the work, and all the disadvantages of the real world, and discovered she did not have time for the fun or the fantasy, which would make it palatable. Wendy is lucky. She flies back to reality and finds peace and fulfillment by living her life to the fullest. Not all those who suffer from the Wendy Syndrome are so lucky. Some keep themselves forever in their own Never-Never Land and become a grown-up in a secluded world – overworked and unfulfilled. Can you be a Wendy and feel satisfied? Perhaps — if the adoration of your lost boys is enough Only you can answer that question – is what you are doing now enough of a reward to forfeit a future of friends and varied interests?

Spiritual and religious beliefs often serve as rewards for the good deeds people do. Certainly, generosity of spirit, and devotion, commitment and piety are desirable traits, and your religion and spiritual beliefs certainly help you to struggle and stumble through the dark tunnel by providing a glimmer of light at the end. Your faith represents your own convictions, but strong as it may be, does it eliminate the possibilities of making your present life easier? Again, you need to do your own soul searching to answer this question.

Future tangible rewards, entailing an inheritance or an insurance policy, may be the motivation you envision. Whatever it may be, spiritual peace or material gains, you probably anticipate a reward for all you are doing, payment for services rendered. Perhaps the reward is penance for past sins or deeds, real or imagined; you believe you did something to deserve your present pain and atone for past sins. What are they? Only you know what they are, or think you know, or very likely are not even sure of what they are. All you know is that sometime or somewhere in the past, you did something horrible. Whatever you did creates great guilt and you must repent. Mind you, the key phrase is "real or imagined." The guilt generated by these acts is oppressive, painful, and incapacitating. The only aspirin that relieves the suffering is your self-imposed situation. Relieving pain with more pain sounds like a strange concept, but surprisingly, that's what most of us do.

For example, a child does something "bad" in anger. He throws a stone at the house and breaks a window. Immediately he knows he did something wrong and feels both scared and angry, very uncomfortable feelings. His parent runs out in a rage, scolds the child, and punishes him physically or psychologically, in essence adding pain to his pain. Now that he has suffered twice, he knows he has paid for his misdeeds. As he grows up, the parent becomes incorporated into his own self. He no longer needs someone to run out and say, "You were bad and must be punished," because the internal parent will tell him this. The internal parent may be harsher than the original parent. Unlike the original parent, the inner parent sees not only the bad deed, but the evil thoughts and bad wishes that prompted the act. Our grown-up child now feels that he can assuage guilt by suffering; the more the suffering, the less the guilt. The problem is that the guilt is like a foam rubber ball that you try to stuff in a smaller box. As you try to push the ball in, a part of it always escapes. No matter how much you suffer, you still feel the guilt and try to rid yourself of it by suffering more and more. You keep stuffing away, but you never quite get the ball in the box. You never quite close the lid. Is there a way to solve this vicious cycle? Yes, but it means a great deal of self-examination to uncover the cause of the guilt, forgive yourself and the original parent, and recognize that the parent inside is too cruel.

We now have identified hidden reasons why one continues to stay in a relationship that is often hurtful and harmful. These reasons are not easy to examine, since you have a vested interest in keeping them under wraps. But until you can carefully peel off the coverings, scrutinize and look closely at the underlying "benefits" of your situation, you will remain feeling hopeless and seeing no relief. If you can determine that being locked in is less scary than making new friends, then you can begin to analyze why making friends is so terrifying. What's the worst thing that would happen if you made new friends? What's next to the worst thing? What could you do to prevent these feared things from happening? What would be the good things that could happen? Are your expectations of friendship realistic? What could you say or do that would be so terrible? Is the appraisal of your ability for "friend-making and -keeping" realistic? Hopefully, from this self-cross examination will come a better understanding of your fears. Nebulous and unknown fears become much less frightening when they are taken out of dark corners, dusted off, and hung out to air. But, those fears will dissolve when the sun shines on you, and you can finally bask in the warmth of self-approval.

Chapter 5
The Parasite's Might

Whew – bet you're glad that last chapter is finished! It's really hard to turn over your acts and motives and discover they have another side. Once you gain that insight, you realize that this trip you are on, this trip that is so difficult, dull, and endless does satisfy certain needs. But I am not going to belabor that point again. What I am going to do is examine another facet of the diamond and look at the other member of your partnership.

I have touched briefly on some of the fears and anxieties that besiege your partner, but now it is time to scrutinize them. You may say, "Leave him alone. He can't help himself. He is too weak. He's too helpless to do anything for himself. He's completely dependent on me. Without me, he'd founder; he'd be completely lost; he might even die. Maybe I could help myself but I can't change him."

On the surface, it seems that way. However, your partner is like a parasite. Why? The definition of a parasite (according to *Webster's College Dictionary*) is: "1. an organism that lives on or in a plant or animal from which it receives nutrients. 2. a person who receives support or advantage from another without giving any useful return." Using this definition, you see how he is attached to you, saps your strength, and needs you. BUT – is he weak and helpless? Would he die without you? Parasites need the proper environment to grow and develop. If allowed to grow unhampered in a confined space, the parasite can become stronger, grow, divide, and eventually harm or destroy the host, regardless of size. Dysentery may be started by a few parasites that become armies that devastate the host. Some parasites such as worms can live in your system and cause no fatal harm, but do cause discomfort. It is possible that one can suffer an early death if parasites are allowed to grow, divide, and spread throughout the environment, whether internal or external. In recent years, there has been much talk and research about tiny elements in the environment that can devastate populations. The might of the parasite is real and well-documented. Less widely discussed are the strength of dependency and the tyranny of the weak.

Think of the parents of a newborn infant. The baby is helpless and unable to take care of his simplest needs. But he can cry. One wail is usually sufficient to summon someone to his side. Two wails will probably produce even more attention. Thus, the baby can commandeer adoring adults to cater to his every need. This is normal, natural, and necessary. As the baby grows and becomes more independent, his demands should decrease and he should gradually care for himself to a greater extent. You could say that in that weak and dependent stage, the baby is "tyrannizing" his helpers. That's a strong word to apply to an infant (you might prefer controlling or needy) but actually, whatever you call it, the child is a tyrant who demands that his wishes be granted. By the same token, if older people remain or become weak and dependent, they too can browbeat their helpers by demands for constant attention to both realistic and unrealistic requests.

You may or may not believe that the meek will inherit the earth, but you better believe that if allowed, the meek can rule the roost and your household! Some of these needs are realistic and must be met. The work becomes overwhelming, and the boundaries of needs and demands become blurred. How do you know when that happens?

Well, let's be very specific and look at examples about how dependent people of varying disabilities demonstrate ploys that might be used. The examples are drawn from people who are addicted, mentally handicapped, psychologically impaired, aged, or medically ill.

Example 1:

Your alcoholic partner, Billy, has been through all the usual channels to help his addiction — the traditional therapies, the encounter groups, the expensive dry-out facilities, the not-so-expensive dry-out wards, the halfway houses, and nothing has had a lasting effect. He is weak and helpless, and without you around, he would get rip-roaring drunk, upset his ulcer, start bleeding, and aggravate his colitis and eventually experience DTs or even go into a coma. Therefore, you can't leave him for any length of time. When you are around, he is so sweet and docile. He helps you around the house, he kisses you, he sweet-talks you, and builds model boats (when his hands aren't shaking). But, as soon as you leave the house for a couple of hours, he manages to find a bottle somewhere or cons a neighbor into getting him one, or steals some money from your secret stash, sneaks out, and the binge is on. In fact, at times, even when you are there, this has happened. Come to think of it, though, that was the day you were planning on a shopping trip with Cousin Joan. Once it happened when he knew brother Joe was coming over. Joe would predictably start his pontifical lecture on the evils of gin. Of course, Joe has no weakness. Think about the sequence of events. Does it tell you something? Billy is terrified of being without you. He can't comprehend what will happen without you. Two hours without you will push him over the brink, or more properly, into the drink. But you say, "He has tried to get better and failed." True, but he always knew you would be there for him if he stayed addicted. He is exerting the only power he has – the power of his weakness. "If I get drunk, I get sick, and ergo, she won't leave me." He's right – you won't leave him. However, not because of his weakness but because of the power he wields.

Example 2:

"Surely," you say, "Christine is an exception. She has absolutely no power. She is so retarded that she can't help herself at all." Are you sure? As retarded as Christine is, probably she has learned some skills – she finger feeds herself, she plays with some toys; she may even be toilet trained. She has some control over some things, simple as they might be, and perhaps some you haven't even noticed. Let's pick one — finger feeding herself. She does that very nicely. She likes to pick up the food and clean off the plate. She seems to relish eating. However, one day you decide let her eat by herself while you will use this time to read a new book someone gave you. As you settle down and open the book, all hell breaks loose. Christine's plate is on the floor and food is scattered all over. Christine is infuriated. She's screaming and kicking and flailing her arms every which way. With some difficulty, you calm her down and then clean up the mess. You get another plate and sit with her while she eats. Lo and behold, Christine does relish her food. She feeds herself nicely, cleans off the plate, and beams under your approval. The book? Oh well, maybe you'll find some time to read, perhaps when she goes to sleep. The fly in that ointment is that you are usually so tired, you both hit the sack at the same time. Aha, isn't

that interesting? When did that start? Well, you noticed that Christine goes to sleep much more quickly and easily if she sees you in your nightgown. Otherwise, she screams interminably. Is she displaying weakness or power?

Example 3:

Jonathan is schizophrenic. He graduated from high school an honor student, but barely finished a year of college at the time he became ill. Since then, he has lived with you, not doing much of anything. Usually his symptoms are under control with medication. However, Jon has never forgiven you or the rest of the world for his affliction. So he chooses not to talk to anyone. Generally, you accept this and chat with him, even if he does not respond. True, this seems to be a one-way conversation, but you accept his grunts as answers. However, his brothers do not accept his remaining mute. When they come to call, they badger Jonathan to talk. He will ignore them and the situation becomes so unpleasant that you encourage his brothers not to come too often. As soon as people enter the house, Jonathan plops down in the middle of the living room, seals his lips, and glowers at everyone. Then it starts. Everyone is yelling and arguing and trying to make Jonathan talk. You can't stand the ugliness and nasty goings-on and wish everyone would go home. All this time, Jon sits there with a sardonic leer and tightly sealed lips. It's much better when you and Jon are alone. Have you ever noticed how Jon acts when you suggest that you should have more company? He takes shower after shower and changes his clothes each time. He dirties all the towels and insists on changing sheets on all the beds. Before you know it, you have ten loads of laundry to do, while he sits on the couch and watches TV. What is Jonathan displaying – his weakness or his power?

Example 4:

What about Dad? Dad is nearing eighty and is pretty frail. His hearing is poor, his sight is failing and he has difficulty recalling recent events, even if they happened today. Certainly he qualifies as helpless and weak. Well, let's see. He usually hangs out and waits for you to take care of his needs. He wants what he wants when he wants it, and if he doesn't get it right away, he yells or bangs his cane on the floor. He can walk with a walker, but refuses to use one. He has resisted all the aids you have suggested to help him hear better or see more clearly. Although you can't always get him to the bathroom in time, he refuses to wear adult diapers. There aren't many things he can do except watch TV. He turns the volume all the way up so he can hear, and blasts it all day long. You are able to tune it out by this time, but it makes it impossible to hold a conversation with anyone who happens to come in. You can't even talk on the phone while he is watching. You try to turn it down sometimes when you really need to talk to someone, but if you succeed in doing so (by wrestling the remote away from him), he starts to nag and whine or yell. "You are terrible to me, after all I did for you!" He enumerates what he has done over and over and ends by saying, "You won't even let an old man have his only pleasure." He goes on and on until you finally decide it isn't worth the effort and get off the phone or ask your visitor to leave. Often, after you do that, he decides it's time to take a nap. Does he exhibit weakness or power?

Example 5:

Dwight's problem is much different. He is in his late forties. He was a vigorous, high-energy person until two years ago when he had a massive heart attack. After his two complicated heart surgeries, you were told that he could never return to his former life. He was not yet a candidate for heart transplant, and he is adamant about never having one, for reasons you find difficult to fathom. However, he could continue to live indefinitely with minimum stress and limited mobility. At first, he stayed at home and was a househusband, but very quickly, when you were ready to go to work, he started to feel faint and dizzy. He would insist that you go to work, and he would call if he got worse. As soon as you arrived at the office, he would call and beg you to come home, since he felt worse and had twinges of chest pains. Shortly after you got home, the pains would subside and he felt better.

After a while, you decided to stay at home full time. His disability payments were high enough to live on and your job was in jeopardy anyway due to your frequent absences. For a while, the symptoms subsided, but as soon as you tried to take some time for yourself, the pains recurred. Though you may doubt that the pains are real, you cannot risk leaving him in that condition. Also, you take comfort in the fact that your presence has helped him avoid a fatal heart attack. Once again, the question arises, weakness or power?

These examples are not meant to imply that your partner is making deliberate efforts to entrap you. We are all guilty of manipulation at times, sick or well. For the most part, this behavior is meaningful but not necessarily malicious. It is simply a defense on the part of your companion against being left alone, feeling frightened, being ignored, scared, helpless, or angry. It is an effective defense, though not healthy for either of you.

When Billy gets drunk while you are away, you take care of him when you come home. When Christine feels neglected, she makes a mess in her pants to get your attention. It works. You clean her up, comfort her, and play with her. When Mike's silence drives everyone else out of the house, you continue to chatter and watch TV with him. You even bake him treats because you need something to occupy your time, which is after you have finished washing all the laundry he creates. And when Dwight's blood pressure shoots sky-high, you do everything in your power to calm him down and lower the stress. The doctor has warned you that another attack could be fatal. What else can you do but swallow your disappointment at missing the concert and keep him calm?

The power that's being exerted travels the wrong way. The one-way street of strength and power is supposed to go from the strong, who are helping the weak. But, lo and behold, what fuels the power this person has over you? Is it love? Guilt? Helplessness? Dependency? Or neediness? It's all of these, some of these, or even none of these. The point is not what causes these ploys to work, but the fact that they do work. Your helpless partner can pull the strings and you can dance like an obedient puppet. He's conditioned and has conditioned you. The longer this push/pull pattern goes on, the more entrenched it gets. The more you dance, the faster the music. The faster the music, the weaker the person gets; the weaker he becomes, the harder you dance.

Let me illustrate this theory with an example. You are playing a game of checkers with your handicapped son. The doorbell rings, and it's your neighbor come to visit. You tell Bobby you'll continue the game later. He starts rocking and banging his head against the wall. You ask the neighbor to excuse you while you finish the game. She waits patiently till after the game is over, and you start to chat. Bobby feels left out and starts to bang his head again. You tell him to stop and you will play with him later. Instead he bangs his head so hard that he cracks the wall. The neighbor hastily leaves, and you soothe Bobby, rub his head, and resume playing with him. Bobby has reinforced for himself a valuable lesson. Rocking and banging gets attention, in this case loving attention. Sometimes the attention is not so loving. You scream, cry, hit or threaten — but it is still attention. Therefore, the more disruptive the behavior, the more attention he receives. The sicker the drunken spree leaves you, the longer you get fed and pampered. After the drugs wear off and you are hungry and tired, you get a cooked meal and a newly made bed. The more you agitate, the more the blood pressure soars and the more solicitude and attention you get. Even one suffering from brain damage finds that the more confused he seems, the more protected he is. Let me emphasize that these situations are not happening out of maliciousness.

What emerges from these examples is that your helpless partner is utilizing his disabilities in self-destructive ways. He may be getting the support and attention he needs or believes he needs from you. However he is going about it in a way that enhances his weaknesses, rather than augmenting his strengths. Perhaps, early on, you did encourage him to utilize his strengths, but that's a hard job and he didn't want to try. Now you have given up the attempt, but still this behavior is not necessary. You are more than willing to give him attention, and indeed you do. Haven't you devoted your life to him? You have, but to a hungry person, the food in front of him is not enough. Knowing that more is in the kitchen is not enough. Your partner demands all he can get, because the fear of losing you is ever present in his head.

The problem, therefore, is not his weakness, but his strength. Utilizing this strength enables him to control you, by making use of his weakness. If you can acknowledge this, you will be ready to think about ways to channel this strength constructively. By using your partner's strong points in a way that enhances his abilities, rather than reinforcing his disabilities, you will be on a new road — one that will lead to a richer and fuller life for both of you. Specific suggestions will follow in later chapters. ***Be assured that I am not advocating abandoning your partner, nor the abdication of your role.*** What we are suggesting is a shifting of gears, a slowing down of momentum so that you can rethink your trip and head for new vistas.

Chapter 6
The Right of Fight

So now you've done a lot of soul searching and asked yourself some very painful questions. You've gone back to the beginning and reviewed how you started on the course you are presently taking. After struggling through all the questioning and probing and facing honestly what has happened, you may realize now that *you* made the choice – it was not made for you. That is the most important insight you may ever have. Recognizing that your situation from the beginning was a conscious *and* unconscious choice will help you to recognize that change is possible.

The choice you made, however, became clouded as the years went by. The original trip you started on gained momentum and tumbled and turned until you lost control. Like a runaway train the speed distorted the scenery, and though you seem to be going somewhere, the past journey, the present one, and future destinations look the same. Your vision is blurred, the landscape is fuzzy, and the final stop is indistinct.

That's what happened to Jane. Jane, when she was twenty-three years old, worked for a large company and entertained hope of receiving a promotion with more responsibility. Her elderly mother slipped on the ice and broke her hip and elbow. Both were repaired but she found it difficult to get around and certainly could not stay by herself. Jane's siblings (six of them) were scattered all over the country. They all came home to see Mom and decide how to take care of her. Mother vetoed leaving her home and going to any facility that could care for her. Her constant cry was, "I raised six children but six children can't take care of one mother." Strong opinions were expressed about how to proceed.

45

Since Janie lived in the same city, she agreed to take a short family emergency leave while they discussed other options. The siblings all returned home, and despite many conference calls, could not come up with an arrangement that suited all parties. By pooling resources, full-time help was a possibility rejected by Mother. She liked Janie taking care of her. Janie asked for an extension of her leave, but after that was up, she had to resign. She may not have realized it then, but her journey on a one-way track had begun.

You can question why you stayed on the runaway train and come to a conclusion you only had yourself to blame. Not true! You had help along the way. First of all, your own needs kept you rooted to the driver's seat and froze your hands to the controls. Whatever those needs are, good or bad, real or imagined, conscious or unconscious, the caring role you undertook nourished and fed them. Relatives cheering from the sidelines spurred you on and kept on you on track if you tried to stray. Finally, your partner — the one upon whom you've lavished so much care — had a vested interest in feeding your needs.

Now let's return to Jane. As time went on, she became restless. She told her siblings she wanted to go back to work and begged them to help her find a solution. The phone calls heated up the wires. "Just a while longer... Mother does nothing but rave about how good you are to her... Right now I am swamped. Maybe later in the year I can help out... Mother seems much happier since you started staying with her... You really are a super daughter... No one could do a better job." There just did not seem to be any other solution. Obviously, Janie could not leave her mother in the lurch. In fact, if she mentioned trying to arrange for someone else to help her, Mother cried and cried. "How could you even think of letting a stranger help me?" So the years passed and Janie's train sped on and on. She was mired in her role and her train made no stops.

Your story will differ from Janie's, but in essence, something similar happened to you. If you've been honest with yourself and you've pretty much sifted fact from fiction, you are ready for change. A word of caution: Don't be upset if you find yourself feeling uneasy and reluctant to take the first step even though you have gone through the process of self-examination. That's perfectly normal. Change is always accompanied by anxiety and the thought of changing one's lifestyle is mind-boggling. The anxiety is usually the result of conflict. Your conflict revolves around the issue of "I know what I have now. How do I know I will be comfortable or happy when I accomplish the change? Even if my world is constricted – even if my life is dull and hopeless — even if I am stifled and dissatisfied – any other life is an unknown quantity."

Look at Marcie. Marcie's father sustained a back injury on the job and could never return to work. Her mother cared for him for several years, but then she died of a heart attack (probably partly due to the constant care of her angry, disgruntled mate.) Marcie stepped into the caregiving role, and for fifteen years, endured her father's complaints and his abusive attitude. She became discontented and dreamed of having a job and paying for her father's care. After all, he couldn't be more unhappy than he was now. She religiously looked through the want ads and circled promising possibilities. Somehow, she could never follow through. Distasteful as her present role was, she was terrified of having any other. Each time she tried to answer an ad, she hung up the phone or tore up the application. Once, she managed to go for an interview, but left before it took place. She was shaking so badly that she had to run home. There she felt comfortable and safe.

This fear of venturing out is a big concern, and probably puts you into the worst quandary you have ever faced. ***However, remember that you must try to keep your fears under control.*** If the anxiety created by the conflict becomes too overwhelming, you will become psychologically paralyzed and unable to move at all. Recognize that anxiety is normal and natural. Accept it as a signal of change and as an inevitable part of the process, and then move on. If you think back to other milestones, such as going to kindergarten, starting high school, going out on your first date, getting married or whatever big step you were anticipating, you may recognize the sinking, fearful feelings. Chances are, the "something" was not exactly as you dreaded. In fact, it may have turned out pretty good. Try not to allow yourself to ruminate on the "what ifs." You'll never find the answer by sitting in a chair and thinking about it.

Polly had been a secretary before she became her adult son's caregiver. He had been in a car accident that paralyzed him. Of course, she stayed home to be his caregiver. After seven years, despite her love for her son, she became obsessed with the thought of going back to work and hiring a helper. She had been an excellent secretary when she was forced to resign, and thought it would not be hard to get back into the routine. But every time she mused about this dream, she began to panic. What if her skills were rusty? What if her son deteriorated? What if the hired helper was unreliable? What if she neglected him? What if she couldn't manage the new computer technology? All of these possibilities overwhelmed and beleaguered her. In her eyes, going back to work presented too many obstacles. If she could be honest with herself, she could see that fear of a new life was the real hurdle.

You too will be paralyzed if you get stuck in the dire possibilities. Never trying to take steps will leave you in the same position. Thinking, planning, and anticipating problems are part of the process. But beware of stopping at that point. For example, someone can spend a long time in therapy figuring out why he is afraid to get into an elevator. After a while, he finally understands the reasons, but still climbs the stairs. He is not on the way to a "cure" until he takes that first elevator ride – even if it is only a one-story ride. After that, he is on his way to becoming an elevator cowboy. Think it out – plan the details –but then **you must act.**

Another cause of anxiety is "suppose I make mistakes?" No one sets out to make mistakes and no one wants to, but we all do. Making the mistake is not the most important issue. What you learn from the mistake and how you deal with it is of prime significance. If you look at mistakes as failures, you will give up. If you look at them as irrevocable, you will feel guilty – and then give up. Mistakes, like most events in life, are not embedded in stone. They can be used as learning experiences. You can review the process that led you to the error and then incorporate your new learning into future acts.

Zoe's mother made a mistake. She left her retarded child with a sitter for the first time. She thought she had carefully planned this venture. She told the sitter exactly what to do and exactly how long she planned to be gone. She spent a lot of time preparing Zoe for her absence. When she returned an hour later, she found Zoe screaming and banging her head – the room in a shambles – and the sitter tearful and wringing her hands. Mother's initial reaction was that all her fears had come true. "I knew this would happen and never again will I leave!" But then, she remembered that mistakes are inevitable and she needed to scrutinize what happened to make things go awry. After she calmed down both her daughter and the sitter, she sat down with the sitter and reviewed step by step what transpired. Things went along okay until the sitter gave her milk and cookies. It seems that she put the milk in the blue cup and Zoe *only drinks milk in the Superman cup. Her mother realized she must keep a more detailed log of Zoe's activities and write down step-by-step procedures if she was to successfully prove to Zoe that she can be lovingly cared for by someone else while Mom is away.*

The routine of taking care of your charge is so engraved in your brain that you don't realize how many details you take care of automatically. So you made a mistake, you learn from it, and you trudge on. Will you feel guilty about a troublesome incident? Probably you will, but you have had guilt feelings before and you will have them again. It's inevitable, not insurmountable. Guilt is real phenomenon when one <u>deliberately</u> does something that brings pain or bad consequences to another. Guilt is not reasonable or acceptable because you planned something that happens not to work. That can happen even when plans are carefully laid out. But certainly you can try to anticipate all exigencies.

You may wonder if you will be totally happy if and when you achieve the major changes in your lifestyle and the changes in the relationship with your partner. It's doubtful that that will be the case. Every change in life is accompanied by some sadness. Remember that the relationship you have had with your partner has satisfied certain critical needs. Perhaps you will have outgrown those needs, but the remembrance remains. It reminds one of the fond recollections of the "good old days." Does one really want to live in the horse and buggy days again? Does one really want to experience again the pre-television, movies, DVD, electronic devices, cell phones era? Life is not only more complicated but much more comfortable than the "good old days." Whatever your own "good old days" encompassed, you will remember them as happy and uncomplicated. You may romanticize those times. We are blessed with selective memories and often our memories select the satisfying parts as the only reality. So expect that changes will bring some sadness.

Growing up has very bittersweet moments. Most mothers dream of the day their youngster goes off to school – a red-letter day for the child and a measure of freedom for the mom. However, when the day finally arrives, most moms are overwhelmed with tears (some shed, some not) at the sight of their youngster trudging into the classroom. In fact, often the child is more composed than his mom. To her, though, the beginning of school days means that babyhood is over. She thinks not of the drudgery of diapers and formulas and potty training, but of the joys of having an infant in her arms. The baby who was so dependent on her will now have other important figures in his life. The mixed feelings this event brings about are part of life itself.

The changes you will make will also trigger feelings of loss and a desire to retain the present. You will need to remind yourself, again and again, of your goals, and acknowledge that your old relationship did not bring you the fulfillment you know you deserve.

In addition to your own anxiety, you will be the target of the fears and anxieties of others. Your relatives, who have been cheering you on for years, will now be frightened of how the changes in your life will affect them. They are comfortable with your sacrifices and will tend to keep things as they are. They will not want to rock the boat and will apprehensively watch your attempts to make your partner more independent and less reliant on you. They will predict dire outcomes and try to discourage you in both subtle and unsubtle ways. You may not be able to rely on their encouragement, and must plan on drawing on your own inner resources for strength and perseverance.

The key words are "Do not overreact." Overreaction leads to discouragement. You have a long, steep staircase to climb. The trick is to take it slow and easy, one step at a time. If you do slip, chances are that you will only slide back a step or two – not the whole flight of stairs. The damage done by your wrongdoing will be less than your fear, if you can take it in stride. Don't be like Chicken Little, who believed the whole sky was falling down when a nut from a tree hit him on his head.

On the other hand, make sure your steps are small and well thought out. The temptation to overshoot the mark, to be too ambitious, or to bite off more than you can chew — is fraught with danger. The mountain may be formidable, but you do not have to climb it all at once. Small goals make the climb much easier, and if you should falter, the backward slide is not as great. Remember the tortoise and the hare. That race was not won by speed and not when the sprinter was overconfident. Instead, slow and steady was the better approach, and in the long run, decided the race.

At times, you may become discouraged and wonder if what you are trying to accomplish is worth the struggle. When that happens, try to untangle yourself from the situation. Step back so you can see the whole picture. Museums provide benches for that purpose. You may need to use that bench. Fantasize that the picture you see of yourself and your partner are two other people in the same position. Pretend that the caregiver is your cousin or your friend or someone else you admire and love. Suppose the partner is their son, husband, mother, or other needy person caught in the same trap. How would you see that situation if you were outside looking in? Or fantasize it's a TV show you're watching. What would you're reaction be? Would you see it as noble or would you see it as disappointing or even unacceptable? By disengaging yourself using that ploy, you might recognize that more independence for both of you may be much more desirable. When you are enmeshed in the scenario, it's difficult to see a positive ending. Try pretending to be the observer instead of the participant long enough to gain a perspective of where you have been and where you are trying to go.

Chapter 7

Moving On

In the previous chapters, I have been encouraging you to be introspective and try to discover the reasons why you have become a full-time, no time for anything else caregiver. During this process, you have unearthed some feelings and motives that help keep you on this path. Now that you have this insight, what can you do about it? Can you take positive steps that will challenge and overcome obstacles that are preventing you from leading a more fulfilling life? You can, and the purpose of this chapter is to offer suggestions on ways to respond to the insights you uncovered. There are no magic remedies, only suggestions of steps you can take that will head you in that direction.

Guilt is a major issue in the acceptance of any commitment that affects our lives. We all have plenty of guilt but, mindful of the burden you carry, there is a strong likelihood you incorporated more than your share. As I pointed out before, a reasonable amount of guilt keeps one out of trouble and helps one avoid past mistakes. Only people who have antisocial personality disorders never feel guilt. Unable to experience guilt and feel remorse, they can continue to commit crimes or exhibit other disruptive behavior. But this is far from your persona. Your excess feelings of guilt were a factor that led you into this bind. So following the guidelines outlined in Chapter 1, you diligently tried to discover the events that gave birth to your overwhelming feelings.

Your analysis led you back to your childhood. You clearly remember one occasion. You did something you knew was "bad" or "forbidden."

There were consequences you did not want to accept, so you kept silent. Someone else was blamed and you didn't own up.

The result? Remorse set in and the guilt became firmly embedded in your emotional makeup. You may only occasionally think about the incident, but the embarrassment and the shame is always a part of you. The guilt lives on, but you can't change what happened. You can't even confess or atone for it now. Does that mean you are forever stuck with the guilt? No, it only means that you have to forgive yourself. Perhaps you should have come forward then, but you didn't. You were young; you were afraid and upset by the probable consequences. Does that excuse you? No, but it explains why you kept quiet. Contrary to what you think, you did not get away scot-free. Your self-imposed punishment was forever living with the guilt engendered by the memory. It has lasted, unconsciously, all these years. Is that shameful behavior worth all that negative energy? Don't you think the time has come to realize what's done is done and nothing can change it? You may relive the incident in your mind but that doesn't change the ending. Only you can do that. It's your memory and you can change the ending by hugging yourself and saying "It's okay, honey, forget about it. Everybody else has."

Perhaps your guilt stems not from something you did, but from something you hoped would happen and it did. Your father dropped dead, your brother was seriously injured, and your teacher lost her job. The magical reasoning of early childhood would embrace this as reality. "I made it happen." Believing that as a small child is normal. Believing it as an older child means your thinking is not mature. Holding that belief as an adult is plain foolish. Thoughts of anger are normal. Casting an evil eye is superstition. In the real world, wishes do not equate deeds. Connecting your angry thoughts to bad situations is an exercise in futility. The truth is, your father had a heart attack, your brother rode his bike into a tree, and your teacher was fired for hitting a kid. You have been suffering from guilt all these years, feeling responsible for these calamities. Look at the facts. Your thoughts were only in your mind. Even if you said them out loud, they were only words. Think logically and lift that load off your back. Release that guilt. Feel the relief.

Here's an illustration from my own life. My mother had been an excellent pianist in her youth, but I never heard her play. When I asked her why, she told me that I was in my high chair and she heard me scream from the next room. Running to see what happened, she fell, hurt her elbow, and could not play anymore. My guilt went ballistic. I was certain that I was responsible for my mother's lost career. We were both grandmas when I finally related this tale to my older sister, and she exclaimed, "That's not true! I was there. Mother dropped a pencil and tripped on it. You had nothing to do with it." Wow. All these years I thought I was to blame. When I thought more about the incident, I realized that it didn't matter which version was true. If I was in a high chair, I was just a baby doing what babies do, screaming for attention. Her falling was her fault, not mine. Not playing the piano again was her choice, not mine. My burden of guilt had been nurtured and kept alive for fifty years.

Thinking about childhood incidents from an adult's point of view may change your outlook also. Recognizing that words do not equal action may change your perception. Accepting that as truth will help you to let go of some of the guilt. Though the details may be burnt into your brain, you now have a chance to recognize that your old feelings are exaggerated, and forgive yourself. Even if you still think the guilt is valid, even if you did do that horrible deed, carrying the excess baggage won't change the facts. What is done is done and even if you can't forget what happened, you need to forgive yourself and move on.

Another possibility is that your guilt is founded, not in the act itself, but in how somebody important to you perceived it. If your behavior was repeatedly admonished and followed by words such as "you should be ashamed of yourself," you begin to believe everything you do is inherently evil. You walk around with this cloud of shame hovering over you. Soon, innocuous deeds became shameful and create guilt. There is still time to grasp the idea that your mother (or whoever said this) had no foundation for always saying, "Shame on you." Why did she say this? What was her motive? Was she trying to teach you to be good? Who knows? You may never know, but use your adult reasoning. You know you could not have been bad constantly. You were conditioned to think that way. It's time to "recondition yourself," and see those "shameful" deeds in a realistic light.

Of course, the possibility exists that the person you wronged is still around so you can confess. This may lessen your guilt whether you are forgiven or not. The only way to lighten the burden of guilt is to stop holding onto it. Let it go. Whatever you did is not worth all these years of retribution. Your guilt may not be related to any event. Maybe you felt guilty because you didn't like someone or snubbed someone, or hurt his feelings. That's the "I shouldn't have" guilt. We also have the "survivor guilt." That may be the aftermath of a catastrophe that caused severe injury to others, but you survived unscathed. The horror of the experience and witnessing the fate of others can engender the notion that "I don't deserve to be saved. Others no different from me perished." This was a common phenomenon of many Holocaust survivors and survivors of major catastrophes, as the Oklahoma City bombing and the destruction of the World Trade Center. Those are biggies, but an automobile accident or a fire can cause similar guilt. The rationale for that judgment is based on your emotional response to the experience. "I must have done something reprehensible to be spared."

Being the favored one in a family or school may seem like a blessing but it's not always a boon. Your "undeserved lime_ight" or the extra attention you receive may cause guilt, especially if you feel the resentment of other family members or classmates. They may say "It's unfair" and you may believe it.

An unorthodox view is to think of guilt as emotional debts. These debts may stem from "bad" deeds, forbidden feelings, or failed expectations. They are interfering with your current life. Since you can't afford to pay them, you could go into "guilt bankruptcy" and clear the slate. You need to truly believe that you cannot atone for past failures or past deeds. You must truly begin to believe that whatever you did or think you did was not that bad. Do not allow unresolved guilt flavor your life now. Don't allow others to use your guilt to exploit you.

Allowing such exploitation is probably a product of your low self-esteem. Self-esteem, like guilt, has its roots in the past. Looking at your family history and status you were assigned may lead you to some interesting revelations concerning your present situation. Think back. What position did you play on the family team? Were you the smart one, the dumb one, the klutz, the athlete, the helper, the pretty one, or the troublemaker? How were you characterized? Did your position make you feel important or inferior? Was it deserved?

If you will bear with me, I'll use another one of own life experiences. My role was that of the family klutz. All my other sterling features took a back seat. I dropped everything, tripped over my own feet, was deplorable in sports, and couldn't even learn to ride a two-wheeler. I felt inept and inferior, especially as I was the last kid to be picked for the team. It was easier to develop activities that were more academic than physical. Despite my lack of athletic prowess, I grew up and went to college, got married and had a child. For some reason or other, when she was two years old, I took her to the ophthalmologist. On a whim, since

I could not recall having my eyes checked in ages, I had scheduled an appointment for myself as well. Much to my surprise, he told me that I had good vision in both eyes, but due to a muscle imbalance, I could only use one eye at a time. Though I alternated the use of my eyes, I could not focus them together. Without three-dimensional vision, I couldn't judge distance, which explained why my racquet never connected to the ball. Instead of being upset, I was elated and burst into the apartment shouting, "I'm not a klutz. I have a visual problem." My clumsiness was vindicated and my self-esteem shot upward.

Clumsiness can be related to any number of physiological deficiencies or late development of coordination. Therefore, "Be more careful" or "Watch where you're going" won't solve your problem. However, the result of this deficiency has its toll on your self-esteem. In my case, since I had no problem with reading or other intellectual pursuits, there was no apparent reason for my "dropsy." I was jeered at unmercifully. (Many siblings seem to have a corner on the market of teasing). Being ridiculed puts you on the low end of the totem pole. You need to assess your own position in your family and remember how it affected your relationship with other family members. Were you pitied, protected, or ridiculed or all of the above depending upon which family member was with you at the time? Though we like to think we outgrow childish resentment, anger, or pity towards others, we don't. We just learn to hide it better. The feelings are hidden, not gone, and really have an effect on handling "helpful" advice from family members. Remember, I talked earlier about distant relatives telling you how to handle your partner. They pass judgment on your care and always have helpful advice. How do you respond to those conversations? Regardless of the way you responded in the past, there are several other approaches. Here are a few of them.

1. Tell them to shut up (though you may use more colorful phrases).
2. Bring up old complaints like "You're always picking on me". This hasn't worked in the past and probably won't work now.
3. Sniffle and say "I'm doing my best."
4. Express your anger and point out "If you think you can do a better job, take her yourself."
5. Pretend enthusiasm and say "What a great idea. Why didn't I think of that?"
6. Just hang up.

7. Say "ah huh" and cry privately after you hang up, feeling completely inept and unloved or scream in frustration and anger.

Before you settle on any of these responses, or other provocative or pitiful ones you can think of, reflect carefully about the relationship you want to maintain or build with them. An angry response will push them away or provoke a fight that neither of you wins. If your purpose is to sever or sour the relationship, take your choice of the above examples. Any of them will eventually lead to a fight that will serve that purpose.

But there is a more practical view. This relative may not be helping you now, but what about the future? Suppose you want more time for your interests and need someone to help. You realize your sister or whoever it might be, is not going to take over, but perhaps you could persuade her to spell you for a weekend or even a week? Maybe she really can't give of her time but does have money. Financial help from any relative, whether it's monthly or in the form of a new TV, will certainly be welcome. In fact, you can initiate the idea of financial help without feeling like a beggar. After all, if they care enough to criticize, they should be willing to lend a hand. So, perhaps antagonism is not the way to go. What can you say that will not be subservient, not be angry, and not sever any hopes of future support? Your answer must to be diplomatic, to say the least. One good ploy is to say you are following doctor's orders. Another is to say, "Ahem, not a bad idea but let me think about it." That last answer implies that you can tell me whatever you want but I am still in control. If you are stoic, you can ignore the advice given and change the subject. Show an interest in what is going on in her life. Refuse to argue. It's hard to fight if the other person won't rise to the occasion. One of the easiest ways to stop a dispute is to say "you're right." Truthful or not, it does put a hole in your adversary's balloon.

Your decision on the response must be based on whether you want to remain friends or continue to be friendly enemies. Maybe that's being an opportunist, but in your position, it's excusable. Of course, your past relationship with that individual may color your decision. Maybe she has teased and tormented you all your life, and help from her is the last thing you want. Perhaps she is older and has always given you friendly advice but never insisted you follow it. Your relations with people — and that includes relatives — doesn't have to remain the same all your life. You are two intelligent adults and given time, have the ability to arrive at an interaction that is more comfortable for both of you. You may be bitter about being the drudge all these years and thus, tend to forget what that particular person meant to you in the past. Try to plan actions ahead of time concerning phone calls that you know will be full of criticism. You take control. Don't let absent people be in charge. This advice may seem vague to you and lack direct instructions. It is and it does. Remember that my purpose is not to give you a set solution. This is a road map with many detours, all of which will take you to your destination. Some are longer. Some are bumpier. You take the ones that feel right to you and fit your style.

Let's not forget the most important relationship of all – the one you have formed with your partner. Chapter 2 defined five different types of interactions between caregiver and care recipient. There are other variations but these broad classifications give us a working definition. Having a balanced partnership (the one labeled Type 3) is the most equitable and lends itself to individual growth. Each person takes some responsibility, and you both try to compromise and co-operate. Some partnerships start that way, or may reach that stage in the normal course of living together. Most of you, if you are reading this book, have not reached that ideal. All the other types are flawed because they are founded on the assigning of blame for the disability. It was your fault, his fault, mostly yours or mostly his. Your view may be skewed or be absolutely right. But remember, your interaction is based on this inequality. Dwelling on blame keeps the wounds raw. All your dealings with your partner are always tinged with either guilt on your part or blame directed at him. So you become bitter, overbearing, controlling, or overprotective, depending on your attitude towards the fault. Your partner responds accordingly. You can direct the blame in any direction, but the disability is in the here and now and your interaction should be based on that. No matter how seriously he is impaired, he must take an active role. That role does not mean he rules the roost — just that he shares some of the responsibility for his behavior. Since you are the stronger and wiser component, you will have to set the course. His contribution may be limited due to his condition, but at least he is contributing. What if you think of your situation as an ongoing drama? There are two main characters and each must perform his part satisfactorily for the play to be a hit. You are the director well as the leading lady, so you want the supporting actor to do a good job. You can't succeed all by yourself (assuming, of course, this is not a one-person show.) You need to collaborate and compromise. Unlike a real play, your drama is not limited to the availability of the theater, and will run for a long time. Whatever the critics say, you know you are both performing in top form.

Aim for consistency in your partnership. Don't laugh at your partner's antics one time and chastise him the next. If he or has chores to do, make sure he or does them, don't do it for him. Whatever he is capable of in terms of his own care and your partnership, he should do and not persuade you to take over. Don't spoon-feed him because it takes too long for him to feed himself. Chances are, he has no pressing business awaiting him . The consistency will encourage more development of his skills and that is a significant component of the caregiving process.

If a power struggle develops, a cooperative relationship is doomed. When you do everything, your power is absolute. He can become a submissive partner and you will have complete sway. He can also initiate the power struggle. He can be rebellious and indulge in disruptive behaviors. He can demand your absolute attention or make a mess of his food. His methods of stripping you of your power may be primitive, but can be effective. If you have to drop everything to clean him up, he has attained a goal.

For a satisfactory caregiving situation, compromises are a key factor. Neither one of you can have absolute control. Shared responsibility is the key. If your share is larger because of his disability, so be it. At least he is participating positively. But it is imperative that he must do what he capable of learning.. Compromising means each of you work together. You doing all of the work by yourself, has placed you in the" no life for yourself" position

Cooperation from your partner sounds like a great idea. At least you think it is a great idea, but your partner may not. After all, he's had a pretty good deal up to now and why should he want to take an active part now? You will first have to convince him that change is a good thing. After you accomplish that, here are two cardinal rules. One, start where he is at, and two, utilize the method that works for him. Convincing people to do something they don't want to do can be accomplished by threats and punishment. It would serve your goal best if that would be your last choice. Other methods might take longer, but they make for a more comfortable relationship. Your

---

motivation techniques can be effective without being harsh. Persuasion, rewards, and coaxing take longer, but cut down on the resentment. Start where he's at in terms of what you want him to do, and make haste slowly. The process of fostering independence is slow and tedious. If you decide it's not worth the effort, you will never change your life. Suppose the first step is for Joey to clean up his room. You could say something like this: "Joey, your room at night is always such a mess. I usually clean it up, but I think you have to learn to help. For tonight, just pick up your shoes and put them in the closet." Using positive reinforcement, you should be able to convince him to do that one task. You up the ante over a period of time until he is doing all the work. This particular example is based on a partner who has limited mental capacity. If your partner is more sophisticated, your approach could be more along the line of "If you help me clean up your room, we'll have time to go for ice cream." If he resorts to crying or tantrum, do whatever you have to do to calm him, except putting the shoes away. He may resist in his usual way, but you must persist in yours. Be quiet but firm. Remember consistency. If you want to achieve it, you must practice it.

This same technique applies to behavior as well. He must know that you will not change your plans for the afternoon, just because he carries on. His alternative to not crying is the promise of something good happening when you get home. If you want your partner to get used to you going out, anticipating a reward may be a good incentive. Again, consistency is the key. Remain calm. He must realize that you will go with or without his permission, and if he cooperates, your return will signify a reward. By the way, a reward does not necessarily mean a tangible object. It can be a game of cards, an extra story, or a special dessert. Agitation stimulates resistance.

This illustration may be incongruous for your companion. The idea behind it is not. Adapt the circumstances and the tasks to his capabilities, but always maintain your calm, be persistent, and practice consistency. Time and patience are on your side. Be prepared for a long-term process. The first step is the hardest. Once your companion realizes you are not kidding, the next step is easier. It may be a long staircase, but you can do it if you keep your goal in mind.

Now it's time to leave the abstract and move to the specifics. The next section of this book puts the emphasis on your partner, his disability, his strengths, and his needs. It offers ideas and suggestions meant to help him control his symptoms and at the same time insure your welfare and safety. There is no way to lump all disabilities and handicaps into one typical group, but we can distinguish broad categories. The people in each category share some characteristics in common. My intent is to use these characterizations to offer suggestions on handling inherent problems. I will describe various handicaps or conditions and suggest techniques to enhance assets and reduce deficits. Even if your partner fits into only one of these categories, I suggest you read them all and extrapolate ideas that you think will be helpful. Your partner may have dual diagnoses. Putting people into categories is imperfect at best. It is possible that your partner's problems may overlap or spill over into another group. Look for methods that you think will work for both of you.

Section Two:
Defining His Issues; Redefining Yours

Chapter 8
Living with Mental Illness

Although chronic mental illness takes many different forms, living with a mentally ill partner does present certain commonalities. For one thing, almost all mentally ill people in the early stages of life seemed okay. Very few people (except in retrospect) are considered psychiatric problems for at least the first few years of life, most not until late teens and some even later. Thus, you probably have memories of your partner as "normal." This colors your relationship, because no matter how often you have been told by a multitude of experts that he will never be cured, you still retain these memories and with them a faint hope that he will be normal again. This hope is often strengthened by the very nature of mental illness. As you have discovered, no one is mentally ill all the time. Sometimes, he seems quite together and good company, even fun to be with. The problem is that just when you are beginning to be lulled into a "maybe things will change" mood, the symptoms reappear and you are back to square one.

Nannette was the oldest child of five children. She was a bright, outgoing, pretty child and did extremely well in elementary school. Teachers thought she was intelligent and charming and the kids vied to play with her. In her second year of high school, things began to fall apart. She seemed preoccupied. Her schoolwork deteriorated and she appeared remote to friends. Her closest friend complained that Nannette was acting mean to her. Then one day, seemingly unprovoked, Nannette started screaming.

Unable to control her behavior, she was taken home. Reluctantly, her parents hospitalized her, and she was diagnosed as suffering from schizophrenia. Nannette did not react well to medication and had many psychotic episodes. Her parents were bewildered by the turn of events, unable to understand how a "perfect child" could become so ill. Despite medications and treatment, her condition remained unchanged. However, her parents kept looking for a cure and throughout her adulthood sent her from one institution to another."

Nannette was a very dramatic case. However, young schizophrenic people will start displaying symptoms, often in the beginning years of college, following a seemingly normal adolescence. Hope that the condition is a temporary phenomenon lingers in family members for a long time.

This hope is fueled by the reality that he is not a "mentally ill person." He is a person who suffers from chronic mental illness. You may think that I'm just splitting hairs, but this statement makes a difference in how you relate to him. Like many chronic conditions, there are remissions and reoccurrences. Only a part of the person is "sick." There are times when he sees things that aren't there, hears voices that only exist in his head, sinks into the depths of despair, withdraws into a corner, or goes on a rampage. But this happens only at times. Even at those times, when the disease seems to be all pervasive, part of him responds in a more normal way. What does that mean to you? It means that he can learn to change or modify his behavior. It means that he can learn to respond to the symptoms of his illness in a more adaptable way. It also means that you can learn to respond to these devastating symptoms in a much more adaptable way – for you as well as for him.

Tommy was a patient on an inpatient psychiatric ward of a large hospital. He was sixteen years old, but no stranger to hospitalizations. One had resulted in a transfer to a long-term state facility, an experience he dreaded to repeat. He was the youngest of three boys, had always been a difficult child, and his parents had totally different ideas of how to control his behavior. He played his mother against his father, and this exacerbated his illness. During his present hospitalization, he had spent most of his time in bed, hiding under the covers. The psychiatric team assigned to his care decided he would have to be transferred to the state facility, since he was not responding to treatment. One of his therapists, not quite convinced he was as helpless as he seemed, approached Tommy, still hiding under his blanket, and told him of the planned transfer. The therapist advised Tommy if he wanted to prevent this from happening, he would have to start getting dressed, go to the day room, and try to participate in some of the activities. Tommy did not respond, but the therapist made a point of repeating this suggestion several times that day. The next morning, Tommy got up and dressed. He stayed in the day room all day and then asked if now he could go home. The therapist told him that he had to continue participating for the team to change the decision. For the next week, until he was discharged, Tommy continued to participate in ward activities. This tactic did not cure his condition, but it did illustrate that the control he had over his behavior could be used to help him adjust to his illness.

Isaac presents another, more complicated example of teaching chronically ill mental patients that their symptoms remain somewhat under control. Isaac was attending a day treatment program. When his voices began to talk to him, his demeanor became quite frightening. He would clench his fists, pace rapidly, and mutter louder and louder. He would call people derogatory names and appear quite menacing. Often, when he was not in program and displayed this behavior, the police picked him up, took him to the emergency room, and more likely than not, he would be hospitalized. He hated being in the hospital, and in one of his calmer sessions, asked the therapist if it were possible to control his behavior. The therapist, who had developed good rapport with him was . encouraged by his question and agreed to try to help. Together they started to pinpoint feelings that triggered these events. He became sensitive to sensations that a "spell" was about to occur. In truth, during these episodes, he was more frightened than frightening, although that was hard for others to believe. If the warning signs surfaced during program hours, he would seek out one of the staff members to try to help him calm down in the privacy of an office. If he was outside, he would look for a less populated area, like a park, where his behavior would not be as conspicuous. It took a lot of conditioning but it worked. He gained some control over his symptoms and although they did not lessen, this control helped him be less susceptible to incarceration.

With these examples as encouragement, I will discuss specific behaviors and suggest techniques for coping with them. Always try to remember that with every symptom of mental illness, there is a point where the symptom of the illness stops and temper or fear takes over. You may have to live with the symptoms and devise ways and means of helping your partner cope with them, but **you do not have to take the abuse. You do not have to be the punching bag – verbally or physically – for your partner's rage, frustration or aggression.** I am not suggesting abandonment for this reason or any other. I am suggesting that if he is unable to set limits, **you must**. Remember that mental illness may not be curable, but it is controllable. There are different ways to control – medication is one, intermittent hospitalization another, an ongoing day hospital program another. You must find a therapist you can both trust. This is an absolute must. You both need to know that professional help is available at all times. Your partner may object to one or all of these procedures. "The medication causes side effects"; "The programs bore me and everyone there is worse than I am"; "That therapist is too old, or too young or too tall or too short." Your job is to ignore the complaints and find ways for him to comply.

I also suggest that another way to control symptoms is by your behavior, which will in turn influence his behavior and help him control his disease. This in no way recommends that you replace his psychotherapist. It only suggests that by making yourself less vulnerable to his disorder and enhancing your own life, you will help him modify his behavior and hopefully enhance his life.

Remember "Jonathan" in Chapter 5? His whole family was held hostage by his refusal to speak. For years, the family tried to make him talk. By not participating, he was in effect holding them hostage. It took a long time before they were able to put in effect the therapist's suggestion that they ignore the silence and not respond to it. When the family was finally able to follow this plan, Jonathan's refusal to speak stopped being an issue. On holidays, the family would eat dinner, and if he chose not to join them, they ignored him and celebrated their holiday around him. Believe me, this was not an easy technique to implement, but once the family was convinced it might work and adhered to the plan, Jonathan realized his mute behavior was not having the desired effect. He began to rejoin the family group, still silent. With no pressure placed on him to speak, he relaxed and the whole family benefited. Notice – this ploy did not make him talk, but speech became a non-issue.

Now let's look at some of the specific problems you may be facing on a fairly regular basis with your partner. The threat of suicide is probably the most difficult behavior that you have to face. First of all, it is hard for a non-suicidal person to understand the depth of the feelings of hopelessness and worthlessness that drive a person to the brink of suicide. This may seem difficult to fathom, but the motivation to kill oneself lies within the person, not without. You may be prone to assume that (1) you are doing something wrong and (2) you can prevent the person from committing the fatal act. Both assumptions are wrong. Despite what he might say, it is not your fault. You are not causing your partner's depression. The cause lies in the feelings of despair and worthlessness he feels. These feelings are, in turn, the result of his intrinsic pathology and his perception of himself and the world around him. These perceptions are based on ancient history, are probably lifelong, and may have little basis in today's reality. Once you recognize this, you may be able to divest yourself from the enormously heavy cloak of responsibility you assume by thinking you are the cause of his threats and that you can prevent him from killing himself if you are with him every waking minute. If he is determined enough, he will find a way to evade the most vigilant watch.

Oliver, a twenty-one-year-old college student, had been displaying suicidal ideation since he was seventeen. He had been in treatment since his first attempt to end his life, and had been hospitalized in a private facility for the past year. After he was released, he attended weekly group therapy. He revealed in a group session that he was tired of living and would like to jump off the roof. The group was properly agitated by this and urged the therapist to rehospitalize him. For several reasons, this did not happen but Oliver seemed more relaxed and made plans to return to college. He did, and seemed to be doing well. Eight months later, Oliver drove to a nearby city, checked into a hotel, and overdosed on pills.

Tess, thirty-two years old, had a long history of depression and suicidal ideation. She had made one suicide attempt ten years ago. Since then, she had been stabilized on medication and living in a supervised apartment setting. One of the stipulations of the residence was attending a day program. One day, while talking to her counselor in the program, she said in an offhand manner that she really was tired of living this way. Because of her history, she was immediately taken to the psychiatric walk-in clinic. After talking to her regular psychiatrist, the clinic sent her to see him. She insisted that she did not mean to kill herself and had no plan. She added that her sisters were coming to visit that evening, so she would not be alone. The psychiatrist decided to allow her to return to her apartment. She agreed to see him the next day and made an appointment. That evening, while her relatives were visiting, she suddenly ran to the window and jumped out. The program, the clinic, and the psychiatrist all tried to claim blame for her action. In truth, the blame belonged to Tess and nobody else.

Both these stories illustrate that it is difficult to prevent suicide when someone is bent on ending his life. Even professionals can make an error in judgment and believe the patient is not in imminent danger. Of course you can and should take reasonable precautions. If he is actively exhibiting suicidal symptoms, it is reasonable to be sure a plethora of pills are not handy or that sharp implements are not lying around, begging to be used. Respond to his feelings and don't devalue his sense of loneliness and despair. Empathy, not sympathy, is the key word. **Above all, do not try to deal with it alone.** Inform his therapist what is going on, and be particularly alert to delusions and voices that urge him to act. In all situations, while being empathetic, let him know that you will do everything in your power to prevent him from killing himself and this means you will get him to the emergency room immediately if the threat seems serious. Hospitalization is not just a threat. He must know you mean to do it and will call 911 to help you do so. Hospitalizing a person when he is acutely suicidal helps him climb out of the deep valley of despair and allow him to return home better able to cope with his problem. You may eventually learn to distinguish between true suicidal threats and manipulative behavior and react accordingly. If in doubt, always take the threat seriously and consult with his doctor. If hospitalization is indicated, go with it – even if he begs and pleads with you, not to do this to him. You are not doing this to him, but for him. The more he recognizes you will not be swayed, the better he will feel in the long run. (1) He knows you will be firm and do what you think is best, and (2) you care enough to prevent him from killing himself. Don't ever be reluctant to seek help. If his regular therapist is not available, ask the police or take him to the nearest emergency room that has a psychiatric walk-in facility. Research the options in your area now, so that you will be ready to implement emergency procedures if necessary.

Closely allied to suicidal behavior is violent behavior. Here the aggressive feelings are directed outward toward the person he lives with, the person who is closest geographically and emotionally. Threats and verbal abuse can lead to actual physical assault. Your immediate concern is not to allow yourself to be the recipient of your partner's rage. If he picks up a weapon, do not attempt to disarm him – call for help.

Stuart, a counselor in a group day program, noticed that two members of the group, Al and Joe, were having a heated argument. He tried to arbitrate but the hostility between the two men escalated. Al suddenly pulled out a box cutter he had hidden in his clothes. Joe wisely backed away, but Stuart tried to reason with Al. Consumed with rage, he brandished the weapon. When Stuart tried to wrestle it away from him he was slashed in the arm. The blade slit an artery and blood spurted from the wound. Luckily, one of the other counselors did not wait for the reasoning to be effective and had called 911. The police and the ambulance quickly arrived. Al was subdued and Stuart was rushed to the ER. His injury was so serious that he was in danger of dying. Numerous staff meetings had emphasized the folly of reasoning with an aggressive client. Not heeding that warning resulted in a disaster for Stuart and endangered others.

The best defense is strategic withdrawal, not reasoning. Joe acted wisely. Stuart did not. When you see the signs of escalation, **get out of the way as quickly as possible.** Violent and aggressive people tend to worsen if they feel crowded or cornered. So **give him space.** Better the leg of the coffee table is smashed than your leg is broken. When you see the signs of agitation, increased suspiciousness, mutterings, or any other idiosyncratic signs you have discerned through the years, do not try to reason. Stay out of the way. Make sure you both have escape routes, so neither of you can be backed into a corner. Remember the cardinal rule: "Never let him position himself between you and the door." Then – GET HELP! Again, if your partner is subject to impulsiveness and violent behavior, have a game plan ready. Names and numbers should memorized, programmed for speed dialing, or at the very least be posted near the telephone. If you have a cell phone, program in the numbers and carry the phone with you. Above all, try to maintain your calm. Disturbed people pick up "vibes" readily, and if he senses you are afraid of him, it only intensifies his own fear of losing control. Often your partner is more afraid of his aggressive impulses than you think. Despite his threats of wanting to hurt you, he is often terrified that he will. Sounds like a paradox, but fear of losing you is still paramount. Thus, it is comforting for him to know that you are intent on protecting him from being the victim of his rage. If you placate him or give into his demands, you are only empowering him with very dangerous ways of satisfying his needs. His threats will become more and more frightening, more and more violent, and eventually may result in disaster.

How can you prevent him from acting out his impulses? The best advice is for you to utilize a consistent pattern of getting out of his range and calling in the troops. You cannot and should not try to control someone who is irrationally out of control. Let people who are trained to do so, subdue him. When he is calmed down and more rational, you will be able to relate to him rationally and discuss what happened. If you consistently follow this pattern, your partner will understand that you will not permit yourself to be hurt or permit him to completely lose control. I'm not suggesting that this response will be an easy, smooth operation, because in fact it may not work. But you need to try. The knowledge that you are firm and consistent should in all probability act as a deterrent rather than a precipitant to violent behavior. Before the situation escalates to this level, however, you may try to keep the peace. If not, call 911. You know your partner better than anyone else, and you can learn to recognize the harbingers of rage. It varies with each individual, but behavior does have a pattern. If you observe closely, you may discern which events are leading to an outburst, and recognize the signs of his irritation. Unusual, frustrating, or upsetting events should be a first clue. We all react to irritating circumstances. Some react adaptively and some in a maladaptive manner. The chances are that your emotionally handicapped partner will have a maladaptive response. He may initially withdraw or become agitated, sleep more or sleep less, eat more or eat less, mutter to himself, or pace the floor, become morose or become loud, reject you or cling closer. Any or several of these behaviors signify that a change is taking place. Heed the warnings and try to acknowledge his feelings. If he is reluctant to share his thoughts or feelings with you, do not insist. At the risk of repeating myself, do not corner him. Allow him space to escape or explode by himself. Don't be an audience and don't put yourself between him and his escape route. Allow yourself room to maneuver. Call his therapist when early signs appear.

Above all, remain calm and determined not to be attacked. By the way, although I have used the masculine pronouns throughout, you should be aware that your female partner could be just as menacing and violent as a male. Don't allow gender to sway you from acting appropriately. It may make you a little squeamish to see your female partner being subdued by the police, but her swings and bites are just as devastating as a male counterpart. A weapon in her hands is as deadly as a weapon in his.

Once your partner has been physically restrained and probably medicated, you can deal with the problems that precipitated the outburst. Remember to pay heed to hints, clues, cues, and your own intuition regarding potential violent behavior. Consult with your psychiatrist about the use of medication either before or after the outburst.

You will also find delusions embedded and hard to handle. One reason is that non-psychotic people find it difficult to understand delusional thinking and bizarre ideation. Additionally, delusions cannot be reasoned away. You know what is happening is not rational, but your partner does not. How can you fathom that someone you live with believes that people come in at night through the closet and steal things? How can someone possibly think that people on TV are giving him secret messages that are often scary? Or how can you understand that he hears voices you can't hear speaking to him? Delusions vary from person to person, but do have some features in common. They are very real to the individual and in a bizarre way, explain his world to him. For example, a common delusion that older people have clarifies for them why things they thought they put away are not where they are supposed to be. Rather than face the terrifying prospect of senility and memory loss, the person believes that someone sneaks in and steals the missing object. This person may have a key, or walk through the locked door or slither in through the walls and hide in the closet. However it happens, in his mind, someone comes in and steals prized possessions – money, bankbooks, jewelry, clothes, etc. Sometimes the delusion becomes more focused and a particular person will be designated as the tormentor, such as a neighbor or a landlord.

Lydia attended a day treatment program faithfully and participated enthusiastically in all the activities. She often spoke about her extended family that she claimed lived in her room at the residence. The family consisted of siblings, aunts, uncles, and cousins. She reported that every morning when she locked the door, the family ascended to the ceiling and stayed there until she came home. As soon as she opened the door, they all descended from the hiding place and spent the evening with her. Her story never deviated. Staff believed that this rather large, happy family existed to protect her from more frightening or threatening experiences.

Delusions frequently take a persecutory flavor and lead one to believe that he will be the victim of evil forces. Therefore, ne must be constantly on the alert and aware of all the devices these forces have at their disposal. With the plethora of electronic devices in today's world, it is even easier now then ever before to imagine that electronic sensors are hidden around the house or implanted in one's body. Rituals may be devised to keep the evil forces at bay.

Joey fashioned a helmet from aluminum foil, which acted as a barrier against dangerous forces. He wore it constantly and if a fellow patient would grab it, he would howl in deep distress until it was either returned or he could fashion a replacement.

The theory that these evil forces are one's own aggressive impulses may be an analytical explanation for you, but will not decrease your partner's belief these enemies exist and wish to destroy him.

Mrs. Gold has not left her apartment for many years. All of her necessities are delivered and left by the door. She would only allow her current social worker to enter. Her apartment was covered with plastic wrap. Her bed literally had a canopy of plastic with an opening she could climb through to sleep. She explained that her neighbors upstairs made electronic devices that would destroy her if the plastic were not in place. She also had every drain covered to protect her from the chemicals her downstairs neighbor pumped in. The delusions would disappear if one could persuade her to take medication. She inevitably stopped taking the pills and the delusions would return in full force.

Sometimes the delusions are grandiose and the individual believes he is a supernatural or famous person —Napoleon, Caesar, Superman, or perhaps Satan. In that role, he possesses mysterious strengths or powers to ward off the danger. Whatever form the delusion takes, the important fact for you to remember is that it has no basis in reality. The other indelible fact is that you will never prove to the person that enemies exist only in his mind. Hallucinations, which are sensory in nature, are equally as stubborn. You cannot dispel hallucinations, nor can you explain them. Anti-psychotic medication may help by controlling the thought disorder, or by reducing it to a manageable size. These are powerful medications and frequently have side effects, which many people find disagreeable. Because of these side effects, patients often stop taking the meds and the delusions return.

Your partner may have to learn to cope with the delusions and hallucinations. He does this by recognizing early symptoms and containing the behavior in an acceptable way. For instance, he may continue to hear voices telling him what to do, but he doesn't have to listen to the message or act on the command. You may point out to him that he doesn't always listen to you or do what you ask him to, so perhaps he can try react the same way to his voices. He may think bizarre thoughts, but can learn that expressing them to strangers outside will only provoke ridicule or avoidance. You can help him structure reality and understand that when he is in the throes of these delusions, he will not respond to reason. You can tell him that you know he hears the voices, but you don't, nor do other people. Therefore when he responds to these voices in public, people do not understand and may even be frightened by his actions. He cannot make the delusions go away but he can try not to respond to them. This approach will, in the long run, prove helpful. It is not helpful to tell him not to think crazy thoughts, or argue with him regarding the delusions or agree with him that his delusions are real.

Phobias, like delusions, will not respond to reason. If your partner is afraid to eat foods that come from cans, you cannot convince him that such food is safe to eat. Saying that the can is rustproof or that botulism is rare or that you eat canned food and don't get sick will not relieve his anxiety, nor permit him to change his mind. It is important, that he knows you do not share his phobia and that they will not affect your lifestyle. If your partner refuses to take the elevator up to the doctor's office, let him walk up the stairs while you ride in the elevator and meet him at the door of the office. This helps reinforce the fact that his phobic reaction is due to his own anxiety and does not reflect yours. Don't stop eating tuna because he refuses it, or stay in the house because he is afraid to leave. Fear of the outside is one of the hardest phobias to deal with since it is so restrictive. Not eating certain foods limits your diet, but agoraphobia (fear of the outside) limits your life. If your partner cannot step out of the house without having a panic attack, you should make every effort to find a therapist who will make house calls.

This is not far-fetched. Contact your local mental health agency for referrals to agencies or practitioners who are willing to treat patients at home. Other sources are medical or psychiatric associations and state, county, or local associations of social workers or psychologists. If all these sources fail, you may have to go through the phone book under these categories and call individuals. Since psychotherapists are licensed differently in different states, ask for credentials. The individual you select should be either a board certified psychiatrist, a certified Ph.D. psychologist, or a certified social worker with a M.S.W. from a recognized school. A legitimate psychotherapist will be gratified if you ask to see his credentials, and should be happy to oblige. If the person becomes evasive or indignant at the request, assume he is not qualified. The fact that he does not want to produce credentials is his problem. You are entitled to know that you and your partner are receiving appropriate professional help.

There are many organizations that will help you deal with your problems with your emotionally handicapped partner. Not-for-profit agencies and self-help groups will provide information and resources for counseling, rehabilitation day programs, or financial problems arising from his illness. Your partner may be entitled to SSI benefits and you should make inquiries at your local Social Security office. These disability benefits may entitle him to Medicaid benefits that might help pay for his therapy or day treatment programs. Day programs or lounge programs not only offer help to your partner, but also offer you much-needed respite time. State vocational rehabilitation agencies may help you find suitable programs for socialization or training. Self-help organizations have many different names in different parts of the country: Parents of Mentally Impaired Adults, Schizophrenia Associations, Families and Friends of the Mentally Ill, Concerned Citizens, to name a few. Your local or state mental health association should be a good resource for you in terms of locating an appropriate group. Another resource would be the social work department of your local hospital or local mental health clinic. Take advantage of these groups. You need all the help you can get.

Remember that changing behavior is a slow and laborious process for anyone and especially for someone whose thought processes are disturbed or distorted. Firmness, patience, and consistency are key attributes to keep in mind.

Analyze behavior that you feel could be changed to make life more livable for both of you. Enlisting your partner's cooperation to achieve this goal may be the hardest step to take. Use all your wiles and the hope of a more palatable life for him. After you identify the behaviors you think should be changed, break it down into small steps and work on those steps slowly and consistently. For example, if your partner is afraid to talk to people, start off by just asking him to say "Hello" to a friend or neighbor. Then add "How are you?" to the task. Work up to a brief sentence about the weather. Then try to get a five-minute conversation going. The concept is gradual change

– nothing dramatic. You will never fell an oak tree with one swipe of an axe. You need many blows, each one penetrating a little deeper before the tree is chopped down. Engrained behavior needs to be chipped away bit by bit. You should not become your partner's therapist, but you can become a true partner in helping him overcome disturbing and handicapping "excess baggage" behavior.

If behavior modification works, you and your partner can live together more confidently. Remember, you are entitled to have a life of your own. You should be able go out with friends or take a vacation. You have the right to satisfaction in your life. Helping your partner get better control of his emotional symptoms is a step towards that goal.

Chapter 9
Living With the Frail Elderly

"The frail elderly" is a term we use when talking about older folks who can no longer manage on their own and need some care and supervision. Many elderly people stay vigorous, active, and healthy throughout their lives. They may live to an advanced age and continue to be intellectually sharp and able to pursue their career for as long as they desire.

The frail elderly are not so fortunate and require on going help or supervision. If you are living with an elderly person who falls in that category, you are certainly aware you are in a very complicated situation. A situation that is so complicated, there are no manuals, no road maps, and no recipes to guide you and for very good reasons. Every elderly person has a long history behind him, a history of his own accomplishments and disappointments and a history of his relationships, with you in particular and a whole host of people in general. He has a personality that has been molded and solidified throughout the years and has developed a whole repertoire of techniques that have worked for him. At times, it may seem as though you are his parent and as a parent might do, you pamper, coddle, and discipline. At other times it may seem as though you are living with a tyrant, an ogre, ten feet tall and twice as fierce. Unlike children though, one cannot chart the growth or decline of an elderly person. The decline might start at age sixty or seventy or eighty or ninety and continue to deteriorate slowly or quickly. This deterioration may not seem apparent at first. However, we do know that all people at some age begin to suffer physical deterioration in different areas. This deterioration may or may not be apparent to the observer. However, the worsening of one's health may act like an eddy or a whirlpool and radiate behavior based on adaptation to (or denial of) the physical loss. Sometimes you may experience or observe a combination of both.

Sophie is an example of both adaptation and denial. She was always a proud woman. She had been the mainstay of her family of origin as well as her own brood. She had no patience for "whiners" and felt her frailties were her own business. She knew that her vision was poor, but did not want to find out why. She suffered dizzy spells and frequent bouts of arthritic pain. As usual, she was stoic and told herself that everyone had minor signs of aging. She also ignored the lump she felt in her breast. She said nothing to her children since she knew they would be alarmed and try to get her to see the doctor. She refused to slow down her pace and continued to drive to the store, shop, and clean her apartment. This way of life worked for her until the day she missed a stop sign and was involved in an accident. Fortunately, all parties suffered only minor injuries, but since she caused the accident and seemed confused afterwards, the police took her to the hospital. There she was underwent an intense physical examination. Her children were called and were appalled to learn that Mother had hidden the state of her health from all of them.. They insisted the lump in her breast be investigated and removed if necessary, and she receive the proper aftercare. When she went home, under duress, she gave up the keys to her car but insisted on living alone as always. The children soon realized that this would not work, and proceeded to discuss with her options she might consider.

There is no timetable that establishes the speed of deterioration or how it strikes. One person may have excellent hearing but failing sight. Another may have acute vision but develop poor coordination. Someone else may be so deaf he hardly hears but can walk for hours without losing his stride. Some people can capitalize on their strengths to compensate for the losses, but others either will not or cannot try to adapt. They need encouragement to do so and guidance to know how.

Sam had experienced many ups and downs in his life. He always maintained a positive attitude, which helped him weather many a crisis. After he retired, he became an avid reader. It was very disturbing when he noticed his vision was deteriorating. He struggled and strained in an attempt to continue reading. His daughter observed what was happening and made some inquiries. After a discussion with his ophthalmologist, she investigated a low vision center nearby and nagged him to go there with her. He finally consented (under protest) still convinced that sheer willpower was the way to go. To his great astonishment, he found out that many devices were available to help people who are experiencing poor vision. He learned to use those suitable for him, and was introduced to the wide variety of talking books. He would not use them as long as he could still strain himself to read, but it was comforting to know there were other options available.

The one common factor all the elderly share is that as a person ages, his body ages with him. Cells age and organs age, and as they age, they lose elasticity and the ability to revitalize. The outward signs are easy to see. A person's hair starts to thin or turn gray, his skin wrinkles and dries, movement may not be as fluid, and other bodily functions become troublesome. We realize very quickly the dulling of sensory keenness, diminishing hearing, failing sight, and less sensitive taste buds. These losses occur at different times of life and gradually intensify. Other signs of aging are less visible but eventually apparent. These signs deal with memory and intellectual abilities, and many older people view that possible loss as their worst nightmare.

Rhoda continued to work at her administrative job well past the sixty-five-year retirement age. Her work involved a lot of detail and supervision of a variety of workers. She began to have difficulty finding the right word and often made her point in a roundabout fashion to avoid the lost word. The nagging thought of brain deterioration was intensified every time this happened. She confided this to friends outside of work, and was briefly reassured that they all suffered some degree of word finding. Her greatest fear was that her workers would be aware of this and would cease to respect her. Her pride dictated that she retire despite the fact that her doctor insisted her problem was minor and exacerbated by worry and distraction. She retired with great fanfare at seventy-two, convinced she had worked long enough. She later regretted her decision since her enforced idleness was not the fulfilling experience she expected. The unhappiness and depression that followed proved so devastating that her children, concerned about possible suicide, would not let her live alone.

I'll talk more about memory recall later. Symptoms of lowered mental capacity may be due to any number of causes such as malnutrition, interaction of medications, depression, or lack of stimulation. A physician made aware of the problem should investigate these and other possibilities.

Clearly, your aged partner is like other aged people in many ways and unique in other ways. Like all of the elderly, he has suffered and experienced an overabundance of losses. He has lost his role – that of breadwinner and head of the family, or as homemaker and mainstay of the household. He has lost many of his family members and many friends. Due to real or imagined financial limitations, he worries about the longevity of his savings impinging on his leisure time, and he limits the events he once enjoyed. Most important of all, he has suffered the loss of self-esteem, and unwelcome changes in physical appearance.

Mary was always considered the beauty of the family. She took great pride in this perception and always dressed elegantly. Even on a limited income she would find flattering styles that set off her figure. Her hair was always groomed and styled. As she passed the seventy age mark, she began to be concerned about the wrinkles and drying skin. Although others thought she still looked elegant and young for her age, she saw all the defects. She began to withdraw from former social activities and became a recluse. No amount of reassurance could give back the image she yearned for.

The older person may feel he is no longer worthwhile or important. He acknowledges he is failing, and is unable to stop the process. In many ways he may be as helpless and dependent as a small child. He may have to wear diapers or use a walker or a wheelchair or have to ask someone to read to him. At times he acts like that small child, but more often, he reacts in his own characteristic way to the humiliation, the frustration and the helpless, impotent rage.

Morris was confined to a wheelchair as the result of a stroke. The stroke also affected his physiological system and he was forced to accept the indignities of losing the ability to control his own bodily functions. Morris had always been slightly sarcastic with a wry sense of humor. Now, however, he has lost all inhibitions, the sarcasm turned to insults, and the humor to mocking others. Although he had always liked to take control, he now dominated everyone with his demands and ongoing tirades. All of his irksome traits were exacerbated and impossible to bear.

Harry had a similar stroke. He had always been mild and affable. Friends and family found him easygoing and enjoyed being in his company. After the stroke, Harry became completely compliant. He followed all instructions and submitted quietly to all the indignities forced on him. He seemed more resigned than depressed. Nothing could stir his interests and he became an uncomplaining shell of a man.

There are other scenarios, but the behavior reflects individual reactions to loss. Of course, you can't change the reality of his deficits. You cannot give back to him what he has lost, and most significantly, you cannot make up for the losses either. However, what you can change is how you interact with him and how you react to the changes he is experiencing. Morris and Harry both reacted in a negative way to the same restrictions, but not in the same manner. Others might be morose or depressed. Others may show a false gaiety and make jokes about themselves. I'm not making a value judgment about the reaction – just pointing out how varied it can be.

Since many of the complaints of the elderly center around physical problems and infirmities, it is absolutely essential that the first step is to separate the real ills from the imagined ones. Obviously this entails thorough physical examinations. Many elderly persons resist this strongly. They fear confirming their own suspicions of possible ailments and threatened by a doctor's possible findings. This is a reasonable concern, since a visit to the doctor often results in admonitions to "give up" something desirable – salt, sugar, smoking, coffee, etc. Far more threatening is the fear of hearing that one has the "big C." This euphemism for cancer, popular twenty or thirty years ago, still has an impact on older people, who view cancer as a death sentence.

He also is afraid of learning he has diseases that will incapacitate him more or make him face his own mortality. Ignorance does not prevent the onset, but can be a cushion against reality. However, if you are to help your partner live out his remaining years in the most rewarding way possible, the sorting out of real and imagined ills is essential. Before the trip to the doctor, keep a diary of the complaints. This entails noting the event preceding the most common complaints. For example, does your partner complain of stomach pains after eating certain families of food (milk products, green vegetables or fruit, etc.) Do stomach pains occur after hasty eating, or after exercise or after you have had a disagreement, or served a dinner he didn't like, or if dinner interfered with a favorite TV show or was delayed by unforeseen circumstances? Such a diary might obviously separate manipulative behavior from a troublesome digestive problem. Stomach pains after upsetting events might respond to palliative medications and the information you garner will be of inestimable value to the physician. It might also point out how you play into these situations and give you more clues to a better way of handling them.

This is not to say that symptoms such as chest pains, stomach aches, or headaches should be pooh-poohed just because you've discovered they are more psychological in origin than physiological. Knowing that means you can matter-of-factly reassure your partner that these pains are real but not serious. Consequently, the pains may diminish in importance and you can both move on. As you have no doubt discovered, arguing that his condition is imagined only leads to the more stubborn assertion you are wrong. This can precipitate a power struggle of major proportion. On the other hand, affirming his contention of distress, or being overly sympathetic increases the frequency and the concomitant demand for attention and alleviation.

For example, let's look at this scenario. While you are preparing dinner, the phone rings. It's an old friend and you chat for a long time. Your partner is fretting because dinner will be late and he will miss the first part of his seven o'clock TV program. He grumbles all through dinner, belches, and complains of stomach aches. He then insists that you have poisoned his food. Your response might be:

a) What do you mean I am trying to poison you? I devote my life to you and all you do is complain and berate me.

b) You poor thing — how bad is the pain? I'll get you some warm milk. Maybe I should call the doctor. Who knows? You might be having a heart attack.

c) There's nothing wrong with you. You ate too fast and are just trying to aggravate me.

d) I'm sorry you're not feeling well, but I'm sure if you just relax and enjoy the rest of the meal, you'll feel better. That was May who called and I haven't spoken to her in a long time. Although I knew it meant delaying dinner, I was anxious to catch up on the news. By the way, she asked for you and sent her regards.

The (d) response may not cure or prevent this behavior, but it does show that you recognize the pain, you are reasonably sure it's benign, and you are realize that he was upset by the circumstances. It shows you are concerned but you will not be bullied into either an inappropriate solicitousness or a no-win fight. If the harangue continues, walk away, go into another room, or if necessary out of the house.

Learning to respond this way is obviously not as simple as it sounds. You have a lot of history in your relationship with your relative, whether you are his child, his spouse, his sibling, or other relative. As a child, perhaps you were expected to respect and obey. Arguing was forbidden and an aura of righteousness hung over his words. Possibly he was abusive, verbally or physically. He was the strong one and you were the weakling. If he was your spouse, the scenario may have been different but the final result the same. You now are experiencing a role reversal and you will respond to this reversal in your own characteristic way. You may be saddened, frightened, resentful, or elated by the fact you now have the upper hand. In fact, you may share some or all of these conflicting feelings. It is difficult to see one's childhood or young adulthood hero and model shrink in size and stature and change into a bullying, whining, frightened, or manipulative aged person. However you respond may evoke in you anger, guilt, or shame. If the elderly person happens to be your spouse, it's painful to see one's youthful sweetheart deteriorate in both body and spirit. Thirty or more years of marriage hardly prepares one to suddenly adopt a new role towards one's spouse. Depending on his needs or moods, you may find yourself his puppet, slave, or parent. These are hardly the golden years the two of you envisioned when young, especially if you are lively and vital and your spouse is old and feeble. Mixed with all the conflicting emotions of love, hate, resentment, and nostalgia is an uneasy fear of "Am I next?" Thus, as indicated previously, your responses to the demands, whines, and manipulations are colored by anger, guilt, or even shame. Being ashamed of your partner's demeanor and appearance may restrict you from going out with him, or inviting people to your home.

Having friends to dinner was Ida's favorite way of entertaining. She loved to cook and show off her culinary arts. However, as much as she wants to continue this custom, Harry's behavior gets in the way. He growls at everyone, complains that no one pays attention to him, and spills food all over himself. Swallowing is hard for him, and sometimes he coughs up the food. Ida is ashamed of Harry's behavior and decides no one except herself should be exposed to him.

What may help ease the pain of his behavior is to remember the cause of the changes. They were not by choice, but due to physical deterioration accompanied by mental and emotional collapse. The role you presently adopt is not an old role readjusted but a new role relating to a different personality residing in an old, familiar body. This new personality needs help to adjust to his new self. He needs to learn new responses and new techniques of dealing with this new self. If you can help him achieve a better feeling about himself and renewed independence (even if miniscule) you can help his aging body live in greater peace with a new outlook.

Achieving peace is not easy. Visit any nursing home and you will see a roomful of men and women, mainly stroke victims with severe disabilities. Talking to their relatives will reveal that some of them had been professionals in their own practice or businesspeople in charge of large organizations or companies. Others were skilled craftspeople or held interesting jobs. It is disheartening to see what has happened to them and how hard it is for them to sit on the sidelines, unable to take care of their own basic needs. Even in this depressing atmosphere, the staff — social workers, psychologists and recreation therapists — constantly encourage these bitter, angry, or resigned people to enjoy activities that provide some meaning to the life they are now forced to lead, a life with the limited skills. Staff members who are so involved emanate enthusiasm that is catching, and over time, these men and women do become interested in one activity or another and relate to each other in support groups. We grant you, staff goes home after their shift and has days off. Days off could be a goal for you to work towards. Those times away help you return with new vigor and renewed spirit.

Many feel that living with an aged infirm person is like living with a young child and that senility is a return to babyhood. Although there are similarities, try not to think of him that way. Infantilizing an older person is derogatory and humiliating. It is true that if you think back, you will remember all the steps that you took to teach a child how to become independent and self-reliant. Remembering those techniques may come in handy now. You taught them basic skills and helped them refine them. Your aged partner is not a child but he, too, has to learn new skills to manage his new self. You may have to brush away your old methods of dealing with him and apply new techniques to helping him to learn new tools for living. Try to remember that realistic reassurance when an ordinary complaint is escalated to impending doom is not much different from offering comforting reassurance to a young one that the shadows in the dark are not dreadful monsters. Careful and precise pronunciation for aged, hard-of-hearing ears is as important as clear concise speech for young impressionable ears. Limit-setting for an insecure demanding elder is as necessary as limit-setting for an immature demanding youngster. But unlike children who have a relatively stable and predictable sequence of development, the elderly experience loss of skills with no predictable timetable, and often no ordered sequence. Their capabilities differ from time to time, depending on medication or mood or physical well-being.

This is particularly true when a person suffers from dementia. This condition is caused by gradual deterioration of the brain. Dementia usually starts with forgetting names and words. This in itself is not an unusual phenomenon for most people, especially in the later years. However, dementia becomes more and more debilitating and the person becomes confused, disoriented, and sometimes delusional. The delusions may be an unconscious attempt to make order out of a very disordered world. Thus, when you are accused of stealing something from a drawer, it may be your partner's way of explaining why the sought-for article is not where it is supposed to be. The realization that he put the article in the clothesbasket or the refrigerator is neither bearable nor understandable. It is a reality too painful to face. How do you respond to accusations aimed at you or others? Rule number 1 – never argue back. It's a losing battle, since you will never convince your partner that this is a delusion. Instead, try to reflect the feeling. "You must be frightened to think that someone is coming through the window." "You're angry at me because you think I took your money." "Hearing noises from the people next door is very annoying."

Help avoid the confusion by being very clear and concise. Use visual reminders such as labeling cabinets or red warning tape on hot water or gas jets. A blackboard may be useful to keep track of the days or for reminders. Remember that your partner is having trouble using his thought processes, so use your ingenuity to help him. Employ visual or auditory clues. Keep the day as structured as possible and make the guidelines clear and concise.

Confusion may become worse if the person wanders off. Realizing he is on a strange street and not knowing which way to go may cause even more wandering. Be sure that he is wearing a wrist or ankle bracelet with his name, phone, and address. You can get a medical identification bracelet, which will list all his known medical conditions. If you find he takes the bracelet off, sew nametags with his phone number into his clothes. Without one of these devices, your partner may remain missing because he cannot be identified.

Mr. and Mrs. K. lived in their own apartment. He was demented, but she had a clear mind and was able to keep house, despite her infirmities. When the neighbor came to visit one day, he left the door unlatched. Mr. K. walked outside, and before his wife realized he was gone, he was nowhere in sight. A frantic search ensued, but he was nowhere in the neighborhood. The family called the police and the search continued. Several days went by, and the family was sure he was ill or hurt or perhaps dead. Two weeks after his wandering started, he was located in a hospital. He was listed as a "John Doe." Family and police had called all the nearby hospitals, including this one, but somehow he had fallen through the cracks. With this possibility in mind, it is certainly is worth the effort to sew in nametags or devise some method of identification that cannot be easily discarded.

We have not, in this discussion, differentiated between Alzheimer's disease and dementia due to other causes. Your doctor must make that determination. There are medications to help control the symptoms and to calm the agitation. The medications for the deterioration will vary according to the diagnosis. Therefore, don't just attribute the confusion to "old age." Get medical advice as soon as the symptoms become apparent.

You may have heard a lot about elder abuse. This is a very real problem. The abusers may be family, neighbors, or caretakers. You may understand (not condone) how one could lose his cool and be tempted to hit back at a crotchety, cranky, demanding, whining elder. Unfortunately, it happens more than you think. In fact, it is a national problem and agencies specialize in discovering and stopping abuse. It may take the form of financial exploitation, emotional abuse, neglect, or physical harm. Family, friends, or neighbors can be culprits. Scam artists use their wiles on the elderly with much success. This topic can be and is the subject of many articles and books, but I am not looking at it as a primary issue in this book. You should be aware of it, especially if your elderly folks are living alone.

The abuse I wish to address goes in the opposite direction. How much abuse do you take on a daily basis? How often does your partner lash out at you verbally or even physically, using his cane or walker as a weapon? Remember, you are not a punching bag – not for a child, not for a peer, and not for an older person. Limits must be set and when the abuse starts, walk out of the room. If it follows you, walk out of the house. The message will not be lost. Without an audience, abuse loses its sting, and when your partner learns that you won't become riled up or guilty depending on your pattern, he will start being more circumspect. This advice is especially important if the abuse is physical. Get out of range and stay out of the way until the anger dies down

Don't forget that violence can also be self-inflicted as well, perhaps culminating in suicide. Suicide among the elderly is a very real problem and sensible precautions must be taken. Heed all verbal threats of suicide and take them seriously. Listen to veiled threats as well, such as "I'm on my way out"; "Your father wants me in heaven with him"; What's the use of going on?"; or "You'll be sorry when I am gone." Make sure that lethal weapons and drugs are locked up, and if the threats are accompanied with depression, seek mental health help. Help is usually available in many emergency rooms. Other resources would be a mental health clinic or a practitioner. Be aware, however, that mental health coverage under Medicare is limited, and many psychiatrists are not Medicare providers. Most states with Medicaid will cover mental health services if provided by a clinic or hospital or psychiatrist but not always social workers or psychologists. Be sure to investigate this so you will not be unpleasantly surprised by a large bill not covered by insurance.

This brings us to the practical matter of available agencies and services. Big cities usually provide a large scope of geriatric services and agencies. Your local services for the aged, sometimes call AAA (Area Agencies on Aging) are the best source of information. In some of the smaller communities, you will probably have to seek assistance on a county level for available services and entitlements. Amendments to the Social Security Act and the Older Americans Act made funds available on a local level. Thus, services such as senior centers, home health aides, and visiting nurse services are probably available. However, remember that budgetary concerns may limit such services, so you really have to do your research as to availability and eligibility. Look in the phone book under local government listings for an agency such as Social Services, Human Resources, Office of the Aging, or Home Relief. If you cannot find any of these listings in your town, look under county listings. If you are still having difficulty locating services, check with the social services department of your local hospital or local family agency. You could try asking your doctor, who may be able to steer you in the right direction. Computer literate folks may have luck finding what they need on the Internet, probably searching on the state's Web site.

Once you have checked on entitlements, you might find that your partner is eligible for Supplemental Security Increment (SSI) or benefits for Medicaid or prescription plans from the state or from pharmaceutical companies. Knowing where you stand financially will help you plan out strategies for extra intervention. If your partner is financially secure, this may not be a problem. However, this may become a problem if your partner becomes afflicted with a debilitating illness, mental or physical, that may eventually require extensive nursing services. The best advice in that case is to see a lawyer before incompetence sets in, or later if necessary. Legal procedures such as power of attorney or guardianship are complicated and should be instituted by legal personnel to insure the best possible care for your partner, and an equitable financial arrangement for yourself. Your local Bar Association should be able to help you find a lawyer versed in geriatric legal problems. Your local Alzheimer's association may also be helpful with advice and resources. Include in your papers a health proxy or living will, whichever is legal in your state.

If possible, have your partner's health needs cared for by a geriatric specialist. Of course, if he has had the same doctor for twenty years, you would probably to seek his advice concerning such care. Great strides have been made in understanding the interactions of medications, and health conditions that the elderly are prone to have. Be aware of both the good and the ill effects. Often, confusion or dizziness may be caused by the wrong medication or too much medication. Just as you might have your child cared for by a pediatrician for his special needs, you should consider a geriatrician for your elderly partner. This may not be available in small towns, but most medical school-affiliated hospitals or other teaching medical centers have a geriatric unit attached to them on either an inpatient or outpatient basis. That also could be a source of private practitioners.

Be sure that if you do obtain special services, such as a homemaker or respite care, that you take full advantage of the opportunity to leave the house and do something for yourself, whether it be shopping, theater, movie, or even long solitary walks. Don't hover around to check up or help. Homemakers will tend to be patient with their charge when your patience has been worn thin. Respite care is just that, services provided so that you can get a rest from your chores.

If your partner is mobile, search out and utilize senior centers, whether it be once a week or every day. Don't forget that he needs companionship other than you, and a senior center can provide a listener, a card player, lunch, and other activities. If every day is not available, take whatever you can get, as often as you can for your own sake as well as his. One last word — time is of the essence. You may have to make haste slowly, and don't blow it by proposing too much too fast. You and your partner have been locked together for a long time. He will resist change and you may have to be devious in coaxing him to take advantage of services other than yours. Remember that change is scary for both of you and each step you take may have to be broken down into many mincing steps. The idea may be introduced and then dropped. Casual references to the proposed change may be the approach for a while, such as, "They opened the new senior center in the old school building. I wonder what they did to fix it up," or "I talked to Josephine today. She couldn't talk long because she was taking her father to the senior center," or "The paper mentions a trip sponsored by the senior center," and so on. Once the interest has been fueled, an off-hand reference to a visit might be made. If you do meet resistance, try to acknowledge it by shrugging in a noncommittal way. Don't press or argue, because you may lose completely. Use your knowledge of your partner to pique his interest and curiosity in any activity you believe will help him lead a richer life. Save your firm, no-nonsense stance for activities necessary for his health or for the enrichment of your life.

The final step is to be aware that the time may come when you can no longer care for your partner at home. A nursing home may have to be considered. There are no absolute rules or guidelines to make that decision. It is based on many factors.

One of these factors is when the physician recommends it because his nursing and monitoring needs are too complicated to do at home. Violent and assaultive behavior is certainly an indication that custodial care is necessary. Extreme confusion can become unmanageable in a home situation. An indication of this is that once you have "confusion-proofed the home" such as pulling off the gas knobs, turning the hot water down to avoid burning of fragile skin, locked up all the medications, and your partner is still finding ways to hurt himself, your vigilance is not enough. Be aware that being a Samaritan becomes foolish when you are courting disaster to your own well-being and your partner's on a daily basis. Living in constant fear for your own safety and his is a strong indication that it is time to start the process for nursing home placement. This step must be taken, and there is no reason for you to feel ashamed or guilty. You have done all you can do to keep him at home, and probably more than you should have done.

Chapter 10
Living with a Mentally Challenged Person

The term "mentally challenged," formerly called mental retardation, covers a large territory. The person's problem may only mean he has difficulty learning academic material and finds it hard to display suitable behavior. This is a relatively mild type of the disorder. The range of disability is extensive. Loosely, according to severity, the definitions may be called moderately, severely, or profoundly impaired. All of these conditions may be complicated by neurological impairment, hearing impairment, visual impairment, or ambulatory impairment. Down's syndrome is in a category by itself, because the facial features and body build — prominent characteristics of children with this disorder — look strikingly alike. It can be determined that the fetus has this disorder while in the uterus and is apparent at birth. However, all people with Down's syndrome are not alike in all ways. Like any other population, ability to learn differs as well as personality. Lifespan has lengthened enormously through the advances in medical science At one time forty or fifty years ago, pneumonia was a serious problem and contributed to an early death. As a result, you rarely saw a person with Down's syndrome as a middle aged or elderly person. Today you do. Thus, like all other populations, retarded or not, they experience the aging process and the problems that accompany it.

As previously stated, this disability covers a vast territory and I will, in all probability, only scratch the surface of it. However, as the partner and/or caretaker of someone who is living the experience, you most likely are aware of his particular condition and its consequences. If you are not, it's time for you to find out! Knowledge of the disability he suffers is of major importance to both of you. The extent of his particular problem is significant in devising ways that will help him live with it. It also determines how you can adjust to it. There are many ways of learning about his particular problem, starting with his doctor and extending to counselors, organizations that advocate for this population, and of course, the Internet. Be cautious in your use of the Internet. As previously stated, the Internet can serve as a font of knowledge and support. If you are computer literate, you have already learned it can be a source of relevant information. But keep in mind, you may also find misinformation. If you happen to latch onto inaccurate information, it may cause more harm than good. Like all other research, you have to know from whence these gems of wisdom are derived. It is, however, a helpful starting place for finding others in your same predicament and sharing experiences. You may learn how others expand their horizons. The computer is not the only source of finding a suitable support group. The organizations devoted to mental retardation are a good starting point.

Because of the vast scope of mental retardation, methods of contending with it cannot be easily categorized. However, the same is true of other categories we discussed, and like those discussions, the best we can come up with are guidelines. Remember, our focus is how to help your partner be more independent so that you can entertain the hope of more self-satisfaction in your life. His quality of life will also improve if you reach your goal. Of course, it is possible that the extent of his disability is such that little more can be done to increase his independence. If that is so, you will have to move on to other supplementary care.

Let us assume that your partner has been through the proper education and training that is available for someone with his type of disability. The extent of this training depends a great deal on where you live. Big cities will provide more choices than small towns. Small towns may have to turn to county levels of education, and other opportunities. However, knowing your partner has been through the educational process, you may assume or have been told that he has reached his potential and that more coaching would be unfruitful. You think you are justified in this belief, because all the professionals have told you that he has gone as far as he can go in terms of self-care. It's reasonable to assume that, but I'm not sure it is completely accurate. So are you willing to try a little experiment? If it works, you might be pleasantly surprised. If it doesn't, you will know that more independence is not possible. What I propose is that you initiate an exercise that may be very tedious and detailed. You will not be able to complete this exercise in one day. But after all, no one is going to evaluate your pace. So be slow and careful.

As you go through the day with your partner, note everything you do to help him, and write it down so you don't forget. I am not kidding when I say *everything in detail*. For example, if he dresses himself in the morning without *any* supervision, you can skip this step. However, that means he picks out his clothes, takes them out of drawers and closets, and puts them on while you are doing something else. If you have any part in this procedure, write it down. Do the same thing concerning his hygiene and breakfast. Does he wash, brush his teeth, and comb his hair alone? Does he get his own place setting, help himself to food, and feed himself? Remember, for this exercise to reflect the true state of affairs, you must be doing something else at the time – reading a book, writing a letter, petting the dog, or otherwise engaged. If this is true, then you still have a blank piece of paper in front of you. Otherwise you have a list of things you do for him, such as put out his clothes, help him with his socks, tie his shoes – well, you get the idea. You may not want to continue this today. That's okay, tomorrow is coming. However long it takes, go through his entire day, listing what your chores are concerning his well-being. Now comes the analysis. Underline what steps he might be able to learn to do for himself, or you can devise a new way to teach him, one that hasn't already been tried. Pick out his shirt? Wash his face? Get his own spoon? Nothing is too insignificant!

Maybe your partner does all his own personal care to both his satisfaction and yours. Okay – then what chores does he do? Which of your chores do you think he might be able to do? Whatever you do during the day, you must bear in mind whether he could do this for you. When you have gone through this list, pick out one thing you do that you would prefer he do for himself. Break this one job into its components. Then try to teach him how to do it step by step.

This seems very time-consuming. Is it necessary? It is if you want him to be even a tad more independent. In the long run, you might learn that he can be taught new skills, even though progress is slow. Remember, whatever he can learn to do (however trivial it might seem) relieves you of a part of your load. It also may give him more self-esteem and pride in his accomplishments.

When we talk about expectations, Debby comes to mind. She was six years old and attending a speech clinic when we met. She had sustained considerable brain damage, including aphasia (difficulty with speech and language) after an accident on the playground. Her injuries did not seem to be serious but she

93

spent the night in the hospital just to make sure everything was under control. Apparently, a blood clot traveled to her brain and she had a stroke. She was the youngest child of four and the only girl. Her mother was heartbroken by the turn of events, and hovered over her, not letting her do anything for herself. After much prodding, Mother went to consult with the local Cerebral Palsy Association to learn some techniques that would enable the youngster to help herself. One idea was to sew Velcro on her coat in place of buttons. Debby was thrilled with the thought of fastening her own coat. For her, it was a step towards what she was able to do pre-stroke. However, every time she was ready to leave the clinic, her mother would invariably say, "Let me do that for you." Debbie's frustration was hampered by her difficulty with speech, but one day she exploded and said "NO! Do self." Mother had no idea how much Debbie wanted to "do self." Through the efforts of the therapist, Debby learned many ways to be independent. Her biggest hurdle was her mother.

This story is not meant to imply that you are hindering your partner's growth. It does illustrate that our own anxiety to take care of a handicapped person may blind us to other potentials. Beverly never even began to develop her potential.

Beverly was moderately retarded. The family was wealthy and she was tutored at home. Her mother treated Beverly as her companion and they spent all their time together. When she was about forty, her mother died, leaving her a large trust fund. The administrators of the fund were concerned about her lack of activity. She sat at home and talked on the telephone for hours – much to the annoyance of distant relatives. Finally, the trustee had her evaluated by a psychologist; he recommended that she should be trained at a sheltered workshop. She was admitted to one but hated it. After a week, she called the psychologist to complain. Her comment was: "Doctor, you know my mother did not want me to be rehabilitated." Any move towards independence was hindered by her mother's need to protect her from the world.

The plan that I have suggested you utilize is founded on a basic principle that you start where your partner is now and go as far as he can go, as fast as he can go or as slow as he has to go. You have been at this level for a long time. It will take patience for him to even want to go further. All of us become comfortable with our way of life and resist change. If you have been doing tasks for him for a number of years, he will see no reason to change. Your challenge then becomes a dual one. He has to learn to want to do more for himself, and then how to do it. These learning tasks can apply to all tasks of daily living. Cooking, gardening, polishing furniture, and other household chores may also become part of his repertoire. Remember that we are discussing a broad spectrum of abilities. Your partner may not be capable of doing complicated tasks, even if you break them down into tiny steps. Your job is not only to teach but also to encourage. Your job is also to assess how far he can go. If you push too fast or too far, his battle for more independence may be a lost cause. If he experiences failure too soon or too often, he will not want to try anymore. You have to believe in your heart that you can help him develop further and expect some resistance and some setbacks. The magic rule may become "slow and steady" and in some instances, slow may be very slow. You will, hopefully, become adept at picking up the slightest degree of improvement and building on it.

Activities of daily living may not be a problem for your partner. That's great, but think of how he can go further in other directions. Can you help him improve his communication? If his speech is poor, can you utilize other ways of helping him express himself? A picture dictionary might be a valuable tool. A letter board is another possibility. Perhaps you can find a computer program that might benefit him. Again, I cannot outline a curriculum, because everyone starts at a different place and progresses at a different pace. The onus is on you to ferret out hidden abilities and to be ingenious about the tools.

Incidentally, although it may seem as though I am stressing only someone who has been handicapped from birth, this is not what I mean to imply. Unfortunately, accidents happen. Illnesses may have neurological consequences and brain damage may be the result. You can apply this technique to people of all ages.

You still think this is all hogwash? How can I suggest that you can teach him things that the professionals could not? I suggest it because I believe that human potential has unlimited possibilities. I suggest it because I think that your living experience with your partner brings you vistas of possible abilities not visible to professionals. I am not implying that professionals, teachers, psychologists, therapists, or social workers are incompetent. A few may be, but most are well trained, have your interests and his interests at heart, and try to discern all latent abilities. The perspective they have, however, is based on a limited amount of time, or in case of teachers, limited span of time. Even though your partner's disability dates from birth, if he has lived at home, you have had many years of twenty-four-hour observation. If he has suffered the disability as a result of accident or illness, you still have a twenty-four-hour-a-day chance to discover possible leads to hidden talents. His psychological makeup has a great deal to do with his ability to learn. Psychological profiles are heavily influenced by depression or despair. What he has learned so far was based on his functioning at that time. At this time and this place, he may be more amenable to learning new skills. Factor your own attitude and psychological attributes into the total picture. Are you hopeful? Are you willing to throw yourself into a task that seems impossible? Are you able to transmit to your partner new enthusiasm and hope? Can you be venturesome and inventive? Can you retain your disappointment if things do not go well? You don't want to make matters worse by expecting too much or allowing him to expect too much. Am I asking the impossible? No, just warning you of possible outcomes and trying to assure you that your self-worth is not linked to the results of the experiment.

Here is a story about a father who had faith in his daughter and the belief that she could lead a productive life. Ellen attended special classes in her local school district. She had been diligent through the years and her teachers felt she was progressing at a satisfactory level. Her father disagreed. He felt that she had more potential than was being tapped. Despite objections from the educational team, he withdrew her from school when she was sixteen years old. He owned a small manufacturing plant and during the summer vacations, had often allowed her to go with him to work. She was familiar with the plant and comfortable in her surroundings. Now he began to train her in earnest. She learned to do simple packaging tasks, and with practice, became a productive member of that department. She was extremely proud of her paycheck, and with supervision was able to manage her money. Wait! There is more to this story. Her father, based on his experience with Ellen, hired other handicapped workers. Ellen fell in love with one of the young men. They wanted to get married and both sets of parents agreed to the marriage. With a fair amount of supervision, the young couple managed their salaries and maintained a small apartment. Sounds like a fairy tale? It's a real story of how one father utilized his imagination combined with consistent, patient training.

Now let's get back to you and your chance to try your wings. Have you taken advantage of all the help available in your vicinity? I did discuss arranging for part-time care so you can pursue opportunities for your growth. Support groups for family members and caregivers offer suggestions based on practical experience. These groups may be part of the mental retardation or neurologically impaired organizations, or they may be self-initiated. These organizations raise money for outreach programs and research. They also publicize knowledge about the disabilities they represent. Learn about any recent research that may apply to your partner and check to see if there are new drugs available for agitation and violent outbursts. Don't assume your general practitioner is aware of the latest research. Most professionals try to keep up, read journals, and attend seminars, but your interests are more focused and more personal.

Check for any sheltered workshops, which may have developed in the past few years. Get yourself on mailing lists that track new developments. You will be flooded with brochures and requests for donations, but you can separate the trash from worthwhile information. Throw the former out and file the latter for future follow-up. Check on socialization groups or day treatment programs. Even if the center is not nearby, the drive may be well worth the effort. Investigate group homes, even though you do not want to place your partner now or ever. The knowledge of what's around is important for his well-being as well as your continuous good health.

If you feel that the home training is not working, perhaps the time is ripe to let go. Accept his limitations and allow him to be the best he can. Permit yourself the freedom to pursue new interests. Perhaps his growth is limited, but that should not limit yours. Your plans must include his future as well as yours. Be sure you talk about possible placement possibilities to those who might fall heir to his problems. Give yourself peace of mind about his life, if you should be physically unable to take care of him. You are not immortal, and being mortal means you are vulnerable to age and disablement. You care deeply about your partner despite all the problems, and you should try to insure that his life without you would be as good as it can be. These are not morbid thoughts, just plans for "in case." In the meantime, continue to explore all the new vistas you and your partner can discover.

Chapter 11
Living With a Physically Ill Person

Partners with chronic physical ailments cannot be placed in neat little categories. Lasting disabilities and limitations caused by disease or the impairment of bodily systems are wide-ranging and diverse. Loss of vision or hearing and/or other sensory deficiencies may create much different problems than the lasting results of neurological damage or diseases that leave behind multiple bodily impairments. Failure of essential organs has ramifications in many areas of living. These ramifications are enormous.

Additionally, physical illness may strike at any point in time: when one is a child, teenager, adult, or senior. Each age group reacts differently but shares the same feelings of loss. The psychological reaction may improve with treatment or it may not. Residual damage may be disabling without pain, or it can be painful and disabling. If illness strikes an adult, it may mean giving up a career and/or a vast upheaval of family life. Essentially, any long-term illness means an incredible disruption of a former life. Your partner may become angry, bitter, or resigned. Each attitude creates a different sense of self. The only common principle is that there must be a period when one tries to mourn the lifestyle that is lost, the dreams that are crushed, the interrupted career, the change of role in the family, as well as the loss of health. These mourning periods for both of you go through stages – sadness, anger, withdrawal, resignation, and possibly eventual acceptance. That last stage is the most difficult, and some afflicted people and partners are never able to reach that stage and resolve it. The mourning may be relatively short, long, or prolonged. One of the partners may struggle to accept the inevitable – the other one may not and may remain in stages of anger or depression. As time goes on and the burden seems endless, you or your partner may mourn again for lost opportunities. No loss, human or physical, is put aside forever. Times of grief return and need to be resolved by facing them and dealing with them. Don't push the recurring feelings of loss under the rug.

Stuart was devastated when he was first diagnosed with Parkinson's disease. He raged at himself, his wife, the disease, and basically the whole world. He and his wife went through the mourning period and life settled down. For a few years, Stuart was accepting of his misfortune and at times even "happy." Suddenly, he changed and became isolated and morose. His symptoms had worsened and his wife attributed the depression to the advancing disabilities. That turned out to be only part of his dejection. He learned, through an old friend, that a former colleague had been promoted. It was a position Stuart had been angling for before his illness forced him into retirement. Stuart's feelings about the loss of his career and the blasting of his hopes returned in full force. Once his wife pried these thoughts out of him, she realized that bouts of depression and despair would reoccur.

When disaster strikes, family and friends are usually available and sympathetic, but as limitations of the condition linger and become permanent, they start drifting away. You become the appointed caregiver, whether the partner is your child, your mate, or your parent. When you accept that role, the long saga of interdependency begins. Is this situation different from the other situations we discussed? In many ways it is.

First of all, the onset is sudden. Clues may have been present, but the actual diagnosis clinches the deal. Treatment and/or medications need continual monitoring. Destruction of bodily functions may mean feeding tubes, breathing apparatus, or other mechanical devices. Mobility may be suddenly impaired or extremely limited. Whatever conditions are permanent due to the disease or physiological failure is unexpected and overwhelming for the family and especially the designated caregiver. Caregivers in this situation, unless they have been part of the medical system, have to learn many ways of monitoring their partner's bodily functions. Initially, the caregiver finds the process and the responsibility overpowering.

Josie was a high school teacher. When her husband Jim suddenly had a stroke, she reacted with deep concern. When they were told that he was partially paralyzed and had problems eating, she panicked. She couldn't imagine that they would manage and survive. He went to a rehab facility and that afforded her a reprieve and time to learn how to care for him. When he was about to be discharged, a therapist came to the apartment and ordered the equipment they would need. The realization what life would be like struck home when the equipment arrived – a potty chair, a bath bench, a hospital bed, and a feeding tube. The wheelchair came with him. She was overcome and panicked when she realized what was involved in his daily care. She had to learn to test his sugar, administer insulin, put in his eye drops, measure his blood pressure twice daily, and monitor the feeding tube. She thought to herself, "I'm a high school teacher, not a nurse. I never wanted to be a nurse. How am I going to get through this?" Her love for him, her willpower, and her innate intelligence got her through the initial period. Her duties became routine, although very often she resented her duties and the need to do them. She tried to hide her unhappiness, but her life seemed endless and unrewarding.

Since it is so challenging to categorize this vast realm of disablement, we have made arbitrary divisions and hope you will be able to see yourself and your partner as fitting in one of these groupings or perhaps straddling two.

Three major divisions come to mind. One is the partner who is non-ambulatory; two, the one who is sensory deprived; and three, the person with lifelong disease. The rationale for this grouping is to help you better understand your situation. This understanding is necessary for you to figure out how to lighten your load and hopefully enrich your life. As always, I are talking about behavioral growth, and leave the treatment of the condition to medical personnel. You should discuss with the health care professional whether any of your proposed interventions will have a detrimental effect.

I am deliberately excluding those who are temporarily ill. The reason for this may seem obvious, but I'll state it anyway. Throughout this book, I have discussed long-term commitments. There will be family and personal issues for both of you surrounding your partner's relatively short-term illness or injury. The dramatic difference is that you know that he will eventually return to his former activities. Since you can see light at the end of a tunnel, you be more tolerant of the current blows to your ego. On the other hand, if your partner is permanently disabled, you may feel your life is almost as restricted as his. It is easier to discuss your options if we look at the broad categories. If your partner's problem entails a combination of these factors or is apparently a temporary state, I hope you can extrapolate hints from this discourse that will serve your particular situation.

Let's start with the non-ambulatory person. A person who cannot walk may not be completely non-ambulatory. If he can manage a wheelchair by himself and transfer in and out of the chair and the bed, he is a non-walker but not non-ambulatory. For now, let's look at the partner who needs assistance to get in and out of bed, to transfer to a chair, and cannot maneuver a regular wheelchair. Now, if he a small child or a smallish, skinny adult, this may not pose a serious problem. However, if you are five-foot-two and your partner is over six feet and outweighs you by fifty pounds, it is definitely a problem. It can be done if you learn the proper way to lift him and if the person is able to participate in the process. Even then, he may fall and your only recourse is to call for help. How do you find help in the middle of the night? You call the police. You'll find they not only catch the bad guys, but they will help the good guys. Don't be a hero. If you hurt yourself, remember you both will be in bad straits. Have a list of helpers. Some may be able to lend a hand in the morning, some in the afternoon, and some at night. Take whatever you can get. A full-time helper is great if your wallet can bear the strain. If not, even a part-time worker takes the stress off your back, literally and figuratively. It gives you some free time and even that thought is comforting as you deal with the everyday struggle.

Eddie and Lucy lived in a two-story house. When Eddie was injured and confined to a wheelchair, the two floors became a major problem. They had no way to convert a bedroom downstairs, particularly as the powder room contained no shower. So he stayed upstairs. It was hard on Lucy, as she constantly was running up and down to bring food, take away the tray, help him to the toilet, etc. Eddie did not like being isolated and was loud and vocal about his confinement. Their grown son came to visit and was upset by the living arrangements. He found a nearby nursing home and located a male attendant. He agreed to come before and after his shift and carry Eddie down in the morning and up in the afternoon. Their son paid for his time and told him if he need a second pair of hands, let him know and they would arrange it. The only other thing involved was a second wheelchair. Though the attendant skipped a day or so, for the most part Eddie was near his wife and did not feel so lonely. Of course, this arrangement made it much easier to take care of him. Both profited and certainly the household was a happier place to be, despite Eddie's misfortune.

This story illustrates that the everyday struggle of living may be lightened. If you have not already done so, have a physical therapist pay a visit and assess your needs. Even if you have the requisite equipment, it would be useful to have a physical therapist or nurse show you some tricks of the trade. Perhaps his doctor can prescribe more sessions of therapy. If so, health insurance may pay for it. If not, it is worth the money to have a rehab specialist inspect your home and recommend ways and devices to that overcome some of the difficulties.

Stan suffered a devastating stroke and became extremely angry and obstinate. He would not accept any suggestions, went out only occasionally because of the wheelchair, and spent his time watching home shopping on TV. Helen saw an ad for a motorized scooter and tried to convince him to consider one. He growled "no" and returned to his show. Helen called the company anyway and found out they would bring one for demonstration. She made the arrangement, and once the chair was in the living room, he had to at least watch the demonstration. He showed a spark of interest, despite himself, and the salesman showed him how to use it. When he found out it came with a key to turn the motor on and off and he could steer it any way he wanted to, he consented grumpily to ordering one. The scooter made a world of difference in their lives. He felt more control over his inability to walk and was delighted to realize he could assume once more the job of bringing the groceries home. They would go shopping together and load the packages on his scooter. He even consented to occasional trips to the museum or movies. Helen did not feel as locked in and was relieved of the burden of pushing the chair. His condition did not change, but his attitude improved.

Living with someone so incapacitated is a daunting experience. You are running yourself ragged trying to help him, prepare meals, take care of medication, assist him with his personal care, and so on and so on. No matter how efficient you are, at the end of the day, you are ready to drop. The end of the day does not mean the end of your duties. This is not a nine-to-five job. It's a full-time commitment with no time off, no vacations, and no personal days. You need all of the above, and you need to find ways to get these fringe benefits. Don't be a martyr. Martyrs tend to die young, so give yourself a break. If you truly cannot afford help, then turn to local social service agencies to find out what you are entitled to. Social workers can be quite ingenious as well as knowledgeable. (This statement is somewhat self-serving. If you have read the blurb describing the author, you know she was a social worker at one point of her checkered career.) The social worker can examine your particular situation, and with your cooperation, come up with a service plan that will relieve some of the burden. You need a vacation from your chores periodically, and respite care is one way to make sure your partner is well cared for so you can loll on the beach, climb a mountain, or read a few good books uninterrupted. Respite care is available in some nursing homes or some hospital adjuncts. Your partner may violently object to you taking time off to have some fun. If you can make the arrangements, hold your ground, be unmoved by pleas and tears, and go off for a few days without guilt. You may encounter resentment when you get back, but by now you are familiar with his stubborn ways and know how to deal with him.

If your partner is ambulatory with the aid of a cane or walker, your problems are not less, just different. His ability to get around means he can help himself from the refrigerator, the pantry, or even go to the grocery store. "What can be bad about that?" you ask. Nothing, if your partner willingly adheres to prescribed diets. For example, a non-conforming diabetic who is totally dependent on you to monitor his meals and snacks can lower his sugar level and maintain it. If he is diabetic and does not comply with his dietary restrictions, being ambulatory means he can access and consume a pint of ice cream. Patients who are supposed to lower cholesterol levels will be able to obtain butter, cheese, and other forbidden goodies. You get the picture.

If your partner has dietary restrictions but has lost the ability to get around due to an accident or illness, you may expect tremendous resentment and anger. If the anger is turned outward, you will be the obvious target. If turned inward, you may be dealing with a sullen, silent, passive-aggressive partner. Either way, you are the one dealing with his attitude. If love, patience, and understanding will do the trick, go for it. However if all your tender loving tactics fail, try being firm and confront him with his contrariness. If this does not work, you would be wise to seek professional guidance for him as well as yourself. Chances are, your partner will reject the help. He may have decided "Things are what they are and that's it." You, however, could not only benefit yourself and lessen your own resentment, but at the same time you may learn or devise ways to lessen your partner's rage. As recommended in other situations, support groups and at least part-time help should be considered. If you can't afford any help, perhaps the barter system might work. Use your skills to do something for a neighbor in return for a couple of hours off during the day. When we were young and poor, exchanging babysitting was a common practice. This way, each couple had a chance to see a movie or go to dinner without the dearly beloved but attention-demanding tots. Talk to friends and neighbors. See if you have a talent to do something in exchange for some of her or his time. Crocheting, knitting, repairing broken appliances, or apple pie baking might be your forte but not hers. Do some detective work. Ask questions and find out what would work with whom. Maybe you can find two or more people willing to give you a couple of free hours for a skill that you can do while your partner naps. Relatives who never gave of their time before might be amenable to a couple of hours a week, as long as they can retain their refrain of "being too busy" or "you are so much better than me." Of course, if you are one of the fortunate ones who can afford help, by all means hire someone. Maybe even a teenager will be willing to "partner-sit" for pocket money. If your partner objects (which he probably will), coax, beg, threaten, or simply state it's non-negotiable – which ever approach works for you.

You can apply some of the same practices for the partner with sensory problems. Additionally, if he is blind, there are safety considerations you must find to lessen the chance of his falling while trying to get from room to room. Chances are, you have already taken him to a low-vision or blind training center where he learned compensatory skills. If you haven't, by all means do so now. Being blind, he depends on you to be his reader, but today, talking books are readily available. There are tapes for all kinds of interests, novels, mysteries, etc. If blindness is his only problem, you are probably not as burdened as you would be for a pervasive neurological disease. However, blindness may be the result of other conditions that require you to monitor his needs and insure his well-being. Deafness may not impair the ability to get around, but it limits communication and also requires special training. A person suffering multiple sensory losses will demand all of your time and ingenuity. Try to free yourself a little by seeking the help of others.

Chronic debilitating diseases such as multiple sclerosis (which strikes the young) or Parkinson's disease (which strikes older people) are not only difficult to care for, but are heartbreaking as well. Both of you must deal with the worsening symptoms and disability. The stricken individual must be allowed to do for himself as much as possible, no matter how difficult it is for you to stand by and watch. In fact, you must make him do for himself as much as he can, and encourage his efforts. Again, there are mechanical aids that may make it easier for him. A foam rubber pad under his plate will keep it from slipping as he eats. Special eating utensils are available. An electric wheelchair will be easier than a manual one, and there is a good chance your medical insurance will help pay for it. (Of course, our above-mentioned scooter is also a consideration and some insurance will be willing to cooperate. The company that sells them knows all the tricks.)

Multiple medications administered two or three times a day requires more than your memory to keep track. Even if your memory is phenomenal, your relief person (and if you have paid attention, you have managed to find one) may need devices to keep them straight. Divide the medication into daily doses. You will find several types of containers in the drug store designed for this purpose. However, if the meds must be administered more than once a day, be more creative. Use small plastic cups or other small containers and clearly mark them to correspond to the time prescribed. Egg cartons might be useful for storage. Your ingenuity will figure out what is best for you or anyone else who might give you respite.

Medications tend to be very expensive these days, and insurance pays less and less. Ask his doctor if generic drugs will work. He might even be able to give you samples. Shop around. Surprisingly, drug stores, even chain stores, do not all charge the same price for the same medication. Look for the one that is the least expensive or order from a reliable mail order company. You may save money that can be used for other purposes.

Finally, again I must stress the importance of support groups. Contact the organization that advocates for his specific disease. You can profit from the experiences and the shortcuts devised by other caregivers.

Chapter 12
Living With an Addicted Person

Being the partner of a person addicted to alcohol or drugs is probably one of the most conflicting caretaking of all. The caregiver feels not only the full gamut of guilt and resentment that other caregivers feel, but also experiences shame, anger, sometimes violence, and great fear for the safety and health of the person with whom he is living. Despite all you know about addiction and its hold on the person, you may still feel that he could "abstain" if he wanted to. This notion may persist despite your exposure to counseling or education on the course and causes of addition. The need to satisfy the addiction entails money. It is highly probable that your partner cannot keep a job, or works sporadically. Since he may not have money but cannot satisfy his needs without cash, the solution is borrowing or stealing from any available source. You are most convenient and he may either "borrow" the cash or use coercion to get you to give it to him. The dreaded end result of these addictions is the possibility of death – via his companions, his health, and or the predators who may take advantage of a drunken or drugged state. You are aware that the places he might be frequenting are not conducive to safety, and when he is out, you live in constant fear of a call from the hospital or police. Fueling your anger and ambivalence is the charm your partner exhibits when he is sober and his repentance for any harm he may have done to you. Promises are made and never kept. Your life becomes a seesaw of hope and despair.

A good example of the seesaw pattern caregivers exhibit is the story of Esther and Jack. Jack was her best friend's son. Both his parents died in an auto accident when he was in his early twenties, He was unmarried and living alone. He always had difficulty finding work. He had no training and little ambition (a combination that does not engender success). Esther was a widow and very lonely. She was angry with her children for not coming to see her very often, and depriving her of her grandchildren. Esther and Jack were made for each other. Sure enough, Jack came to visit and broached the idea of moving in for a while "to help her out." When he first came, he cleaned and cooked and shopped and did the laundry. She was completely happy until the day he left the apartment and she realized all her cash went with him. When he came back a few days later, it was clear he had been on a drinking binge. He was contrite and begged for another chance. She thought of all the things he could do for her and acquiesced. Thus, the seesawing began. No matter how many times he stole from her, she took him back. She said she felt sorry for him, and he was good to her sometimes Her friends told her she was weak, and her children told her she was crazy. They did not realize he was satisfying her need for attention, and regardless of the circumstances, welcomed his return home. She would negate the financial abuse, painful as it was. Her answer to her critics was always the same: "His mother was my best friend... I can't throw him out. When he is sober, he is a big help to me."

Your partner also experiences guilt and shame. He realizes when he is sober, that this way of life is damaging for him and devastating for you. He says he wants to stop but is driven by forces beyond his control. He rationalizes that stress forces him into using or drinking, but feels that these pressures are beyond his control. Then again, he may like his addiction and see no reason to stop. After all, "I am only hurting myself and if I choose to do so, that is my choice. Stop worrying about me and I'll do just fine." Companionship is another problem. His old friends (pre-addiction) become frustrated and disappear. The people with whom he drinks or uses only aid and abet him. Often he is in the company of unsavory characters and fear of what they might do is a constant worry for you.

It is a reality that violence may result form his indulgences. Violence aimed at you is his way of controlling you and your money. Nobody deliberately wants to be hurt, but the shame of having someone find out or the fear of what he might do if others interfere keeps you in pain and fear. You also worry if this violence and desire for satisfaction of his habit will lead him into crime or that his companions might injure him.

Mrs. J. has no clue as to when Joey might go on a binge. Sometimes every-thing will seem just fine. He's eating regularly, jokes with her, and helps around the house. Then, she takes a nap and when she wakes, he is gone. Other times he is irritable, argues with everyone (even the TV), and in sudden burst of anger, runs out. Either way, he is gone for some time and returns home dirty, disheveled, and surly. After he sleeps it off, he is contrite and promises to do better. Mrs. J. is so relieved to have him safe at home; she pays no heed to his promises. The cycle starts all over again.

Every addict is an individual, but all share some if not all of the following characteristics. There is a deep feeling of shame despite the bravado, shame about his appearance, shame of his conduct, and shame for failing you. He often feels guilty about hurting you and himself. The guilt is accompanied by depression. True, some of the depression may be organic, due to the persistence of his habits. Some of it may be reactive to his situation. The cycle is set in motion. He drinks to overcome and forget his depressed feelings. Continued addiction brings humiliation and he withdraws from people. He doesn't want to be bothered by anyone who is not sharing his dilemma. He dodges recriminations and attacks before he can be attacked. His enjoyment of life is limited to the times he is high. Coming off the high is dangerous if it leads to thoughts of self-destruction. He may be filled with self-hatred. He may loathe what he is doing, what he is doing to you, and how he has destroyed all his own dreams of life and career. He hates himself for not being able to stop. He hates himself for failing to carry through on treatment programs or self-help groups. As he is begging, borrowing, or stealing to feed his habit, his aggression hides a loathing for what he is doing. If he projects this hatred onto you, he feels you despise him. This will give him the rationalization to continue to deceive you and prey upon you. The catch is he dreads the thought of you abandoning him. You are the one who takes care of him despite his abuse. If you were not there, he would truly be alone in the world. He may enjoy the high, but you are there for the aftermath. You pick up the pieces though he is disheveled, sick, and cranky. His greatest fear, expressed or not, is that one day he'll wake up and you will be gone.

So what is his rationalization for staying on the merry-go-round? He will say that there are too many demands on him. He must indulge in his habit to endure the stresses of life. If things were more peaceful, if he had a good job, if he had his own money, he could abstain. His rationalizations fall apart because even if things are calm for a while, he reenters the cycle.

You think you understand him and his motives, but do you understand your own? You are as shamed by his actions as he is — maybe more so. You try to keep others from knowing about his habits or at least minimizing them. Why do you feel shame? We have to go back to our previous chapters and review the reasons why you are willing to accept the responsibility and the concomitant shame for his actions. You have to review your needs for love and acceptance to start to realize that his habit is not your fault. You know that the responsibility for his actions unfairly rests more on your shoulders than his. If you have been able to absorb and integrate all the factors within you that led you to your present situation, then you know that you are the result of your needs. His problem belongs to him. You are not the reason he continues on his road to self-destruction. More than any other problem partner, the addict will do his best to make you believe it's entirely your fault. It is up to you not to acknowledge it.

Paula was an only child. She was a beautiful woman and a brilliant student, graduating form law school at the top of her class. She shared an office with a friend and seemed to be making a nice living. Her mother was naturally proud of her daughter and bragged about her to anyone who would listen. So, it was a great shock when out of the blue, Paula came to her parents and asked for a large sum of money. When pressed for a reason, she admitted she started taking drugs in college. The stress of starting her own practice increased her need for coke. She owed money to her dealer and he was threatening to "teach her a lesson" if she did not pay him soon. Her parents were appalled but gave her the money on condition she would agree to go to a rehab center. She promised and she went. As soon as the two weeks were up, she was back on drugs. She would go on a tirade and claim she went on drugs because they put too much pressure on her to succeed as a child. If they hadn't pushed her to be the best in her class, she would not feel as inadequate as she does now. It is all their fault that she is in this predicament. As time went on, she found other reasons to blame them. She went into program after program, but never stayed dry for more than a month. By this time, she was living with them. They believed her contention that it was their actions that had put her on this merry-go-round. Their guilt was overwhelming, but guilty or not, they could not bear watching her destroy herself, but they also could not bear the thought of her dying in the street. At least when she did come home they knew she was safe.

While reading that story, there's a good chance you recognized that they were enabling her habit. It's easy to see that in someone else's situation. Take a good look at your own circumstances. Are you enabling his habit? Think carefully and be honest with yourself. What would make you an enabler rather than just his partner? Try to answer the following questions truthfully. Nobody except you will know your answers.

Do you make excuses for him to other people? Do you try to hide his addiction from relatives and friend who do not know about it? Do you leave money in places that he can find? If he takes the money, do you let him know that it is unacceptable or do you ignore it? Do you excuse his abusive behavior because he doesn't realize what he is doing? Do you allow yourself to be a doormat either from love or from fear?

How you answer these questions will determine if you are his enabler. You are the only one who can decide if you want to stop accepting that role. Suppose you decide to stop enabling him, what can you do? For one thing, you should not make money easily available. Make sure the bank knows he cannot access your account. If you suspect he has figured out your PIN numbers, change them. Do not use dates that he would easily remember as the new PIN number. Let him know you will do this because you will not tolerate his thefts. Your money is needed for necessities, like food, rent and clothes. That takes priority. You may incur his rage, so make sure someone is around to protect you and support your position. If it is too overwhelming, go for counseling for yourself, not for him. Nagging <u>him</u> to go into treatment is not effective. Treatment is effective only when he is motivated to change. Your nagging will not make that happen. Reasoning is equally ineffective. There is no harm in trying to reason with him when he is in a receptive mood, but don't be disappointed if it does no good. The bottom line is that you cannot change someone else. You can change only your behavior and indicate you will not condone his.

What do you do about friends and relatives? Some of them will berate you for "not doing anything." The solution they pose is usually "make him stop" or "throw him out." Of course, they have no clear conception of how you can make him stop, short of locking him up and throwing away the key. Throwing him out may be a solution for them, but doesn't work for you. Other helpful ideas are "Call the police"; "Drag him to a rehab facility"; "He won't stop because you put up with it"; "If I were in charge, I would do things differently." Of course, they are not in charge and they will make sure they will never be. How do you respond to them? Be apologetic; agree with them; argue with them; try to prove your approach is the right one; throw a temper tantrum; change the subject; ignore them; throw them out of the house; sic your dog on them? You may be tempted to do all or some of these things. However, friends and relatives are not going to solve things for you. Past history proves that. Perhaps you can tell them politely you will take it under advisement and invite them to leave or leave you alone. Don't make excuses for yourself or for him. Friends and relatives usually turn out to be "advice givers" not "advice implement-ers." You are not obligated to take abuse from them because you haven't solved the problem. The truth is, by yourself you can't make him stop. With his cooperation, you may take the steps to help him, but it needs his cooperation, and if you enlist it, it will still be a long, painful journey for you both.

There are groups in the community that can offer help. Of course the first one to come to mind is the AA type of group. It works for a lot of people, but there is no guarantee it will work for him. Rehab facilities are prolific. Some are private and costly, some are Medicaid sponsored, some are under the aegis of a community agency, and there is no guarantee that rehab will work either. The thing about addicts and rehab is that it is often a revolving door. The addict leaves with all good intentions and plans, which may dissolve as soon as he is back in his own world. If and when he goes back, the attitude is, "Don't give up. Maybe this time it will take hold." And, maybe it will! Many addicts do manage to lose the monkey on their back. It is difficult for them, but it can and does happen.

Despite that last statement, does it sound like I am depicting a gloomy and hopeless future for you both? Perhaps, but don't give up on the idea of groups. At the risk of being redundant, there are many groups for *you* that could offer support for you and suggestions from others who have been in your shoes and maybe still are. You may get ideas from them that might work, but more importantly, you are helping yourself. You may find compassionate people who want to help you deal with both his and your problem. That's all well and good, you say, but I am not a group person. I shrink from other people or become tongue-tied. Listening to other people's problems doesn't make mine go away or even make me feel better. Well, if that's the way you feel, look for an individual counselor – not for him and his problem, but for you and yours. Private counselors are available and some accept insurance. If that is not an option, you could look for a clinic that is sponsored and doesn't need your contribution. A church or hospital or some other local organization often sponsors clinics. It may take some diligent ferreting, but you will find a clinic somehow and somewhere.

Why am I harping on help for you? Because this book is based on the premise that you deserve that help. What about you? Do you have to be either a victim or an enabler? Can you find a way to continue living with your partner without recrimination? Are you addicted to the addict? Do you accept the burden of his problem? Can you be there as a partner and not part of the problem?

You also must realize that as a partner, you are very prone to depression. Who can blame you? Your situation alone can cause depression. However, other things aid and abet your desolation. You have to examine for yourself the factors of guilt, sense of failure, and your need to reform him. You have to think about your life as separate from his, knowing that if you pursue the same course without this examination, there will be little chance of recovering from your depression, from your addiction to him, or ever leading a more fruitful life. Again I urge you, if you have not yet done so, seek the aid of a mental health professional. Fighting depression alone under these circumstances is well-nigh impossible.

Can you accept being your own person as well as a partner? Can you pay heed to your past discussions on your needs and try to understand why you feel trapped and responsible? I am not telling you to desert him. That is your decision and yours alone. What I am suggesting is rereading the first section of this book and seeing how those ideas apply to you and your situation. I repeat that having an addict for a partner is probably the most frustrating of all partnerships. You may and should support him if he tries to reform, but you cannot make him do it and you cannot force him to abstain. You can change your attitude and your behavior, and in some way achieve an independent life of your own. In that process, you need not throw him out or suppress your feelings for him. You can refuse to accept his abuse, physically or psychologically. You can assert yourself and your right to a life not governed by his addiction.

Section Three:
Considering Alternatives

Chapter 13

Be Fair to Homecare

Now the time has come that you know the only way you can have some freedom is by the use of homecare. Someone must be there when you are not and you have exhausted the hope of relatives coming to your aid. However, how can you resort to this? All you have heard are horror stories about homecare workers. "They are lazy. They watch television all day. They bully the client. They steal," etc. Of course there are a few homecare workers who fit some of the categories, even some who fill all of them, and some who are guilty of even more. However, there isn't a profession in the world that doesn't have its bad eggs and black sheep. Homecare workers are not highly paid, have clients who may yell at them or abuse them, and understandably, some may be unhappy about the job in general. The majority of homecare workers are very compassionate and many grow very attached to their charges. Remember, you also have negative feelings about your partner at times, and you have a longstanding relationship. You have to get over the hurdle of believing that these tales of misconduct are the gospel before you can even begin to look seriously for a helper. Let us relate some true stories of devoted workers.

Jessie had been a part-time worker for Mr. M. for the past two years. She had coaxed him into going out more often. She brought a homemade treat with her at least once a week. Mr. M. began to look forward to the times she was on duty. One day when Jessie arrived, she found Mrs. M. unable to get out of bed. She had the flu and was running a high fever. Jessie helped out all day, caring for both of them. The following day, she came again. Mrs. M. thanked her tearfully but explained she had no extra money for additional homecare. Jessie got very upset and said "Don't worry about that. Not everything has to do with money. I'll come every day before or after my other part-time job to prepare food and make sure you have everything you need and I will not even dream of charging you until you recover..

Martha had been helping out with ten-year-old brain-injured Amy, coming twice a week for four hours. Amy was a difficult behavior problem, but Martha worked well with her and they had grown very fond of each other. Amy developed complications and was hospitalized for several weeks. Although Martha had other jobs, she came every day to visit Amy to reassure her that she had not forgotten her.

Daphne arrived one day to find Mrs. K. in tears. It was her husband's birthday and she could do nothing to celebrate it. Daphne pooh-poohed her and spent part of her four-hour shift dressing up Mrs. K. in her best dress, putting makeup on her, and finding a ribbon for her hair. Then, she took her out to find a birthday card. Mrs. K. objected because she had no money. Daphne bought her the card of her choice and said it was her contribution to the event.

I could relate hundreds of stories of compassionate, thoughtful, and devoted homecare workers. But I think you get the picture. Now let's move to the next step. Have you seen homecare workers in action? Do you have any idea of what they are supposed to do? How do you find out?

If you live in a city or town, you have doubtlessly seen wheelchairs on the street. Try talking to the "pusher." He may be a homecare worker and be willing to tell you what he does and why he does it. If you find it difficult to engage a stranger in conversation, just observe. Do you see any cruelty? Do you see any impatience? Make your own survey. True, it is not scientific or broad, but you aren't writing a proposal for a grant. You are only trying to determine if your prejudices hold up in these limited circumstances. You cannot take the homecare route unless you feel it has some chance of success. You need to overcome your reservations, or at least put them aside until you give it a try. Perhaps someone in your support group (we're still pushing) has had good experiences she is willing to share. Get over the hurdle of believing that bad homecare is the gospel, before you even begin to plan.

First and foremost, you need to understand that homecare, if not covered by Medicaid, will run into money. Actually, very few states even have a Medicaid Home Care program. As you know, however, everything about Medicaid and Medicare is currently under great discussion and great controversy. Please keep that in mind while assessing your own accessibility to those funds. It is a good idea to follow the news so you can take advantage of any new favorable decisions. If new regulation will not help you and you can't afford it on your own, it may be time to appeal to other family members for contributions. Remember, you have read all the previous chapters and are now aware of your self-worth and your need to explore your own interests. You realize you will have a better relationship with your partner if you spend some time away from each other. These thoughts should fuel your calls for financial assistance. The money may be an issue for your relatives as well. Be creative. Perhaps siblings and/or children would be willing to each contribute four hours of homecare once a month (or less frequently if you come from a large family). If someone balks, suggest they chalk it up to a birthday gift. It can't hurt to try.

Let us talk a little about the costs of homecare. Why do agencies charge so much? Certainly, the worker doesn't get paid the hourly fee you will pay. The price that the agency quotes you seems very high. However, the homecare industry, like any other business, needs to factor in the costs of operation, which entail more than the wage paid to the worker. Like any other business, they have to pay the normal expenses of clerical help, rent, electricity, office equipment, phone, etc. Disability insurance coverage and workman's compensation are absolute necessities for the survival of the agency. Supervision is provided and someone has to assign the aides and keep track of their hours. Most agencies have a nurse on staff to troubleshoot and provide skilled nursing services if needed. The agency also takes care of social security payments and withholding tax. These additional costs are not only good policy but are required by law. Some, because they work part-time, may not be entitled to sick pay, vacations, and other side benefits. The hourly price, which seems extremely high to you, reflects the costs required to run the agency and, of course, they need to make a profit to stay in business. The advantage to you is that the worker is screened and supervised. A substitute is sent if the worker is ill. You do not have to worry about filing tax reports and insurance.

You also have the option of hiring a freelance worker. You will probably pay her less per hour, since she doesn't have all those expenses, but you are the one who is responsible for reporting wages to the government. You need to consider what could happen if you don't have disability or workman's compensation. If all goes well, nothing will happen. However, if the worker injures herself lifting your partner or slips on the kitchen floor, you may be liable and be uninsured. Most homeowner's policies will not cover someone injured in your home if he is working for you.

You must remember that home care workers are not nurses. For you, that may be a downside. Aides are not allowed to administer medicine or do any of the other monitoring jobs that you regularly perform. They can't test for blood sugar, monitor a feeding tube, take blood pressure, or do anything other than routine custodial care, prepare meals, wash clothes, and do some light housework. The regulations in your state might vary, but on the whole, a homecare worker's job has limitations. In your case, it probably won't be a problem, since you probably are considering a part-time worker and you will still assume charge of the procedures the aide is not allowed to perform.. If you are not available to administer a dose of medication, you will have to devise a plan to solve that issue. That was an important concern in the following vignette.

Mr. S. has both social and medical problems and no family. He was referred to a social work agency that cared for a large clientele of frail, elderly people. He was typical of the folks who either had no family or were estranged from their family. His wife died five year ago, and he had no children or other relatives young enough to help him. He lived by himself in the house he had shared with his wife. At this point, it looked like a disaster area. He refused to allow anyone into his home, and talked to the social worker through the locked door. The social worker was extremely patient and gradually talked him into allowing her entry. The house was filthy. The kitchen was covered with fast food containers, clothes were strewn all over, and the house apparently had not been cleaned since his wife died. He obviously needed help. Talking him into accepting an aide was the first problem. Getting one who was acceptable to him was the next concern. The assigned social worker played a crucial role in convincing him to give it a try. He was badly crippled by arthritis, had difficulty walking, and probably had other medical conditions, which he did not know about or didn't care to discuss. Since he had not seen a doctor in five years, his medical history was a mystery, and as far as he was concerned, would stay just that way. He insisted all was well, and was indignant at the thought of allowing a homecare worker in his house. He said he would lock out anyone assigned to him. The social worker, with an inordinate amount of patience, was able to establish a connection with him, especially when he found out she had lived on the same Caribbean island he came from. Gradually, he trusted her and allowed her to accompany him to the doctor and help him buy much-needed new clothes. He finally agreed to accept help, provided the person could pass muster with him. The homecare agency was very obliging and sent out aides for him to interview. He finally found an aide he liked. The doctor, as a result of the medical examination, prescribed daily medications. Since the aide could not dole it out to him, the social worker called the Visiting Nurse Service. A nurse was assigned to come on a weekly basis to check his vital signs. At that time, she put daily dosages of medication in individual containers. This way the aide was able to remind him when it was time for his meds, and he could administer them himself. As a point of interest, the social worker located an estranged grandson and managed to effect reconciliation. Happy endings are always a delight!

I hope I have not discouraged you with the truth about costs. It is a realistic concern and no one but you can decide if your pocketbook (with or without subsidy) is the way of getting hours of freedom. That being said, let's assume that you have made the decision and have the means to proceed. Let's look at how you can avoid the pitfalls of "bad" aides and find a homecare worker who is a gem. Don't forget the most magnificent of gems needs to be polished and protected. They can't be left in the rough if they are to achieve value. In order to get first-rate care for your partner, you have a lot of work to do. The first step is to investigate the agency before you employ one. The Yellow Pages are a starting place, but you know that the biggest ad does not equal quality. Call the Better Business Bureau and find out if any complaints have been lodged against a particular agency. Learn how many years they have been operating and how much experience the supervisor has. Ask for references. Ask if you might interview the worker and find out if you can easily change workers if you are not satisfied.

The same admonitions apply to self-employed workers. Some homecare workers feel they can do better financially if they operate on their own. Do keep in mind our previous statements about the precautions you need to consider before employing a freelancer. Just as a reminder, the employee should have access to liability insurance. This may not apply to your partner, but remember; disabled people (like everybody else) can become angry and strike out, accidentally or on purpose. You may have insurance that covers a paid worker, but that is not likely. Check so you aren't sorry later on. By the way, a local social service agency is a good source of information. Many agencies have had experience with homecare and can advise you how to proceed. But you still have additional research to do. Chances are, you are interested in a part-time worker. There may be a minimum amount of hours or days that a worker or agency will accept. Some will work half days, some will not. Figure out your needs and financial resources before embarking on this venture or what you may prefer to call your adventure.

So, you have considered all the pros and cons and finally have hired a worker. The worker will arrive with the agency's list of what is acceptable for her to do and what is not. We previously talked about the fact that the aide may not be allowed to administer medication, but can remind your partner that it is time to take it. If you have the meds arranged in dosages and labeled as to time, the worker's job will be easier and her mind at rest about advising the client to take the proper pills. Perhaps a timer would be helpful. Try to make this chore to as accident-free as possible.

Spend time discussing your partner with the worker. It is necessary for you to tell her beforehand his schedule, his quirks, his likes and dislikes. Write down explicitly everything that needs to be done in your absence, and post the list in a prominent place. Answer her questions honestly. You do not want her to be caught by surprise. Planning is everything!

No one can perform a job satisfactorily if not adequately prepared. Part of the preparation is making sure your partner is adequately primed as well. He must also know the extent of her duties and her limitations, assuming he is able to comprehend. If he is very apprehensive the first time, you may assure him that you will pop in a little while later to check on how he's doing. That means that you can't wander far the first day, but it's best to hang out nearby so you can be reassuring if necessary. The timing and extent of your presence is dependent on his anxiety level. You can't overdo it or the whole purpose of having a relief helper is lost. The only caution is to be sure it's his anxiety you are working on and not yours. Deal with your anxiety away from home base.

If you are committed to taking time for "me", you must prepare for some apprehension on your part as well. You can steel yourself with the principle of the "greater good." It may be difficult now, but eventually you will both profit. He will learn not to be completely dependent on your care and you will learn that a refreshed caregiver is a better caregiver.

It is essential that you must have faith in the whole concept of home care. Otherwise it won't work. If you are ambivalent, you will find reasons to discontinue the service. That will put you back in complete control and of course, once again tether you to the caregiving job.

It is really up to you to make sure that doesn't happen. Remember your goal and how long you have worked to take the first step. You have gotten over many hurdles in your history of caregiving and this is just another one. **Whatever you decide to do with your free time, you have the right to do it and enjoy it!**

Chapter 14
What About Day Care?

Day care is a wonderful boon for both the disabled and their partners. There are day care programs for all kinds of problems and all types of disabilities. The emphasis runs the gamut from counseling programs to work programs to social programs to therapeutic programs. Most are geared to a specific population. Some are time-limited and some are for chronic conditions with an open-ended time frame. Actually, it would be hard to improve on the types of programs that have been devised and are effective. Creative people who know the population conceive programs that cater to both general and individual needs. Some stick to tried and true methods, others are more innovative. There is a catch, though — there just aren't enough of them. The waiting lists for admission to some programs are very long. The requirements for admission may be based on school history, medical diagnosis, and past behavior. For example, a history of violence can be a deterrent for group programs. Others will look closely at the past violent behavior and decide they are equipped to handle the problem if it occurs. There are programs designed to change anti-social behavior. In short, it is reasonable to believe that there is a program that will fit your partner's specific need. However, that particular program may be geographically impossible for you to utilize.

The rationalization for specific requirements is to prevent failure and insure success. Successful programs are much easier to fund, and materialistic as it may seem to you, funding is a major issue. This is especially true in the present economic climate when states, cities, and philanthropic organizations are forced to curtail resources. Many programs are designed to cater to the needs of a discrete group of people. If a majority of the participants match this crite-rion, the likelihood of success increases. The rationale is that it's not fair to the square peg to put him into a round hole. This assessment may sound a bit on the sardonic side, but we must admit that there is some validity to the theory. Other professionals contradict this theory by maintaining the curriculum will profit from flexibility. Fortunately, programs do exist with elastic criteria and will accept folks who deviate from the "norm."

Day programs are funded in various ways. Some are dependent on grants from the city or state. Some are subsidized by social service organi-zations, some by religious group, and there are resourceful co-ops formed by concerned next of kin, who may run it while looking for sponsors or seeking backers first.

The demand for day programs began to increase in the 1950s. The cata-lyst was the discovery that chlorpromazine, a newly developed compound, had a soothing effect on surgical patients. From this finding, some psychia-trists deduced the medication might be effective in calming mental patients. Some psychiatrists began to administer the drug to their patients and re-ported successful outcomes. From this beginning, Thorazine was developed and tested in state hospitals for the mentally ill. The tranquilizing effect on uncontrollable patients was startling, and the hospitals administered the medication with enthusiasm. As you would expect, the success of one medi-cation stimulated the development of others, and within a few years, many anti-psychotic medications were on the market and extensively in use. Pa-tients could leave the wards and wander around hospital grounds.

On a personal note, in 1953, when these drugs were proving to be ef-fective, my husband was hired by a state mental health clinic. Housing was tight at that time and the state allotted us an apartment on the grounds of a state hospital until we could find an apartment. Along with young medical residents and families, we lived in a wing of the administrative building. Every sunny day, we watched the attendants bring out a ward full of patients who would all sit in the sun for an hour or two. Because of the medications, many were tranquil and sat quietly. Apparently, some did not respond as well, and we witnessed posturing and unruly behavior. The latter were quickly returned to the wards. Some of the patients enjoyed watching our young children play, and waved to them. The kids always waved back. For many of those patients, it was the first interaction with the outside world that they had experienced for a long time. As depressing as that story may seem now, at that time, it was a miracle that long-term patients were able to tolerate being outside.

Before long, patients taking these drugs could be discharged to the community. Around the same period of time, journalists and social advocates undertook investigations of homes for the retarded and chronically ill. Horror stories were exposed and in the wake of these revelations came public demands for reform. All of these factors led to a concerted attempt to release patients to the community with aftercare and thus lower the population of institutions, which in turn could be smaller and more attentive to the remaining patients. Deinstitutionalization did lower considerably the number of inpatient people with serious problems. However, the second half of the equation, outpatient care, was sorely inadequate. Attending post-care facilities were basically voluntary and had no way to enforce compliance. Many patients were returned to their family or hometown with little more than a small supply of pills, prescriptions for medication, and recommendation of follow-up treatment. Existing clinics were overwhelmed; housing for those without family or with family unwilling to keep them was in limited numbers, and all in all, well-intentioned efforts to allow handicapped people to lead a freer life found many pitfalls.

Day treatment programs became a godsend to people languishing in boarding homes or hotels. Those that catered to this population soon became overloaded. Despite good intentions, it took a long time to formulate programs that could meet the needs of people accustomed to living in institutions.

Here's some more interesting and distressing history. When patients were discharged from state hospitals in large numbers, alternatives were scarce. As previously stated, many, of course, returned to their families. Those who had no family or were not welcome by remaining family were forced to find alternative housing. Dilapidated hotels, either in cities or in rundown resort areas, became home to many. In New York City, a number of old hotels were filed with ex-patients. They were given a tiny room and usually at least one meal was available. They lived on their Supplemental Security Increment checks, which were certainly not large enough for upscale living. The hotels also housed addicted people and ex-prisoners. Mental patients usually stopped going to outpatient clinics and stopped taking medication. Needless to say, this did not make for a safe environment. Managers did try to help them and local social service agencies sent outreach workers who attempted to steer their clients to appropriate clinics. One social service agency devised a program that would attempt to do some minimal training and prepare them for more advanced training facilities. Psychiatrists employed in that program came back from hotel visits both appalled and fascinated by what they found. These young doctors had trained after the advent of psychotropic drugs, and had never seen patients who once were kept on back wards because of uncontrollable behavior. Now, the patients released due to the effects of the medication, without supervision stopped taking the drugs and reverted back to their psychotic stage. The medications at that time controlled psychosis but often had uncomfortable side effects. Many patients stopped the meds because they could not tolerate the side effects. In time, however, these hotels in prime real estate areas were torn down and the guests for the most part ended up on the streets, city shelters, or old nursing homes that provided services reimbursed by state monies, usually Medicaid. In later years, many of these homes were exposed as maintaining horrific environments.

The growth of day programs was stimulated by these conditions and they began to modify programs better designed for the discrete needs of people they wished to serve.

Also, as medical knowledge increased, many people once diagnosed as retarded or disturbed were reassessed as learning disabled, neurotically impaired, autistic, or with other conditions that previously went undetected. Existing programs were not appropriate for many of these types of disorders, and new ones that were more appropriate to their needs were developed. Resources were stretched, and hence, waiting lists.

The mentally challenged, unable to take care of basic needs due in a great part due to lack of training, were usually placed in some kind of caretaking environment — foster homes or group homes — upon discharge from institutions. Some were returned to their families, who demanded that programs be developed to meet extraordinary needs. Emptying state hospitals and state homes was an ever-popular idea and usually a legally mandated one. Finding the proper environment for these patients created other problems. I hasten to add that most of these homes or hospitals tried to find adequate places for both residential and treatment facilities, but good intentions were hampered by the lack of outpatient services.

This is an abbreviated story of the beginning of outpatient treatment for needy clients, and obviously is sketchy at best. As the years went on, more and more programs were developed. Many of the new ones were innovative and therapeutic. Many old ones reevaluated their syllabus.

This is all very interesting, but can it help you? Well, it is comforting to know that programs are designed for people with varying problems.

However, you still face a few problems. One is finding the available programs for your partner's needs. Two is convincing yourself that this is a good idea. Three is convincing your partner that this is a good idea and then implementing the plan.

As usual, you must take into account the difference between the metropolitan areas as opposed to less-populated ones. There are more programs and more diversified ones in the cities, but if you live in a less-populated area, you can probably find several in the county or nearby cities. This may mean that they are not nearby, but if you can solve the transportation problem, it will be well worth the traveling time.

Let's describe programs in general. They are usually developed around the needs of the selected population. Some are structured programs and the client has a schedule of interest groups through the day. Some are sheltered workshops aimed to help those who have the potential to work in a sheltered environment with much supervision. These workshops try to train and graduate their clients to similar work in less sheltered environments. Of course, some clients will never function outside a protective setting, but many can and do. Programs for folks who can function on a higher level will have rehabilitation components that try to arrange for limited placements or future training. Lounge programs are loosely structured and are more like social clubs. Clients follow their own interests but are encouraged to participate in areas such as food preparation.

Let's not forget our elders. Senior centers are for the aged person who is able to mingle and communicate with his peers. Day programs exist for the frail elderly. Many of these are affiliated with hospitals or nursing homes and have the ability to provide some medical monitoring. Some of those centers will accommodate elderly persons who suffer from Alzheimer's disease or other types of dementia, but usually those folks attend groups specially designed for memory disorders.

Persons addicted to alcohol or drugs also have groups focused on their needs. Inpatient detox units are time-limited, but recommend outpatient therapeutic programs as follow-up. Most everyone is familiar with Alcoholics Anonymous and the related groups for family members. Those addicted to drugs have similar groups, though some meetings may include all substance abuse problems.

Okay, you are convinced that attending a day program is a good idea. You investigated your area and surrounding ones and find that they have waiting lists or are not really geared to your partner's problem. What now? Here's another story.

Two women in a relatively small community were caring for demented husbands. Since there was no available program to help them out, they decided to see if they could form one. The first step was to post fliers looking for suitable candidates. After they found several candidates, they went to the local state representative and asked for help. Through her office, they arranged a meeting of those involved with demented spouses and local service agencies. The turnout was much bigger than they expected. Having a politician on your side does add credence to your cause. A committee composed of agencies and spouses and a clergyman were empowered to come up with ideas for the next meeting. In a relatively short time, plans were initiated for a two-day-a-week program, funded by a potpourri of small grants. The time limit was for cost-saving purposes. Without going into the actual details, within six months, the group started. It was so successful that three years later, it expanded to full time and soon was a model for other groups in neighboring vicinities. Two women who desperately needed respite found a way to achieve it for themselves and others.

You, too, could start the ball rolling, if you want some time off and a bonus for your mate. Perhaps utilizing the talents of one of those support groups I keep talking about might be a way to establish something that will meet the needs of you and your partner. Funding may be a hurdle, but part time may be easier than full time. Some of you may remember the co-op nursery schools that young mothers started when nursery schools were at a premium and expensive. You must to tap on all the resources you can think of – churches, local politicos, organizations, colleges, city or county agencies to get help, ideas, and follow-through. Go slow and keep your sights low at first. There's time to expand.

The moral of the story is that if you can't find a ready-made model program; try to tailor one to fit your needs. Remember, you are not alone. There are many people out there with similar problems. Find them and pool your ideas. What one person can't do alone, an interested community may, with more resources, facilitate ideas and make them become a reality.

Chapter 15
Working for the Disabled

You and your partner have lived with his disease or disability for a long time. You know the problems, the heartaches, and the disasters. What can you do about it? How can you help assure a better life for you and yours? Are you willing to join the battle?

People have deviated from the norm since the beginning of time. The Bible discusses many afflictions, such as the blindness of Jacob and the stuttering of Moses. It enjoins children not to desert their elders when they are become old and forget their learning.

For centuries those who were deaf or blind or crippled adapted to society as best they could or were segregated and lived in special institutions. Special schools for educating the blind and deaf were in operation in the United States in the nineteenth century. The "simple-minded" or "crazy" were protected by their families or confined to almshouses or other institutions.

However, as science and medicine became more sophisticated and specialized, broad categories of disorders were sorted out, named, and categorized. Today, knowledge of diseases and debilitating conditions is complex, and diagnosis a complicated art. To help solve the resulting problems of research, new medications, and acceptance by the public, organizations of relatives and other interested people were formed to inform and advocate for each individual condition or disease. Organizations are sources of information, sponsors of support groups and counseling, and money raisers to help their members and advance research, hoping for a cure. The organization advocates in the areas of schooling, transportation, acceptance, and public understanding of the various disabilities.

Telethons, local and national, raise money and consciousness. Pamphlets and booklets are published and distributed. Many publish a monthly or yearly newsletter or magazine. You certainly are aware of the mailings and telemarketing appeals.

Celebrities from all fields have been coming forth to reveal their individual battle with addiction or breast cancer or Parkinson's disease. They talk about struggling to help their own children afflicted with autism or AIDS. No one is immune. Actors, actresses, ball players, political figures, presidents and presidents' wives, movie stars, writers – people from all fields have revealed their problems to the public in an effort to help the cure or elimination of the disease. And it helps. It helps in terms of bringing public attention to problems. It helps raise money. It helps to encourage research. It helps them to accept their own disability, and by accepting it, to fight for a cure. It helps in many ways.

AIDS, alcoholism, drug addiction, breast cancer, Parkinson's, paraplegia, cerebral palsy, Down's syndrome. autism, muscular dystrophy, and multiple sclerosis are only some of the conditions that have celebrities in the forefront. You probably can think of others. Some well-known individuals lend their name to a cause out of interest or by knowing or having friends so afflicted. The reason is not the important issue. The important factor is that people come forth and publicize and help in whatever way they can. Anyone in a wheelchair may engender sympathy, but the same person fighting for his cause inspires respect and tends to get results.

So, how do you help? You may not be a celebrity in the public's eye, but nonetheless you are a celebrity to your family, your partner and friends. Do they always show their respect for you? Perhaps not all the time, but if you are astute, you hear admiration for your courage sneaking in once in a while. You do not have to be a celebrity to become a force in changing the perception and the rights due your partner and yourself.

The Americans with Disabilities Act of 1990, which spells out the rights of disabled employees and the obligation of the employer to implement the necessary facilities for them, is a significant act, since it prohibits discrimination based on disability. It was not the first legislative act to recognize educational and training needs. On a national level, it was preceded by other acts, such as the Rehabilitation Act of 1973 and The Older Americans Act, and other acts modifying and adding to important issues. Individual states have statutes dating back to the 1800s for special educational institutions. All of these regulatory policies and laws were fostered by grass roots organizations long before they reached the halls of Congress or state legislatures.

The job is not over. Despite public interest in the disabled and the advances that have been made, much still needs to be done. You can take an active role and not necessarily on a grand scale. For example, pushing a wheelchair around New York City in the early 1990s meant struggling with many obstacles. Despite laws and regulations, ramps were missing from many street corners. You can just struggle and possibly cuss. But you can do more than that. Those ramps will continue to be neglected if the proper department is not informed or the available money allotted to other repairs. You can make phone calls and write letters to the street maintenance department and ask for repairs. You can call, write, or visit your local political representative and give him a list of obstacles not only of those existing problems in general, but also of others you encounter.

Most public buildings, office buildings, and stores have handicapped entrances. The law mandates this provision of services. Elevators should be available. Most amusement theaters will try to be wheelchair or handicapped accessible or inform the public that they are not. A few try ingenious ways to comply with the regulation. For example, Molly found an unwelcome and distasteful "compliance with the law".

Mollie finally persuaded her wheelchair-bound husband to go to a movie. They decided on one, and she called the theater to ask if the theater was wheelchair accessible. Receiving an affirmative answer, they went to the theater. Upon their arrival, they encountered a flight of stairs. The manager said that the theater had no elevator, but not to worry. They will comply with the promised accessibility. Much to the dismay of the caregiver and the humiliation of her partner, two employees carried the chair and its occupant up a flight of stairs.

This experience thwarted any other thought of movie going. Mollie did not act on the issue; she merely rented videotapes. She had several avenues she could have pursued.

1. Write to the Chamber of Commerce.
2. Complain to the local governing council.
3. Speak to someone at the local organization which advocates for access for the disabled.
4. Write a letter to the editor.
5. Become a member of an organization that represents the disabled in general or your specific problem.
6. Volunteer to help the organization in some way.

Are you getting the idea? Please note that these suggestions center on watchdog agencies, political clout, organizational strength, publicity, and your own participation. If a poor condition is not reported, nothing will be done. If changes are to occur, they usually start on a local level. How do you get started? The first thing you must do is find what services are available and what resources are needed. Do your homework. Look around you and gather information. Then think about your own strengths. What am I good at? What do I like to do? Am I a behind-the-scenes person or do I like to be in the forefront? Strength is in numbers, so look around for a group that seems most likely to advocate for your cause. Talk to others you know in your predicament and see if you can find enough people to form a group or participate in a group that will espouse your cause. As always, your search has to vary by your neighborhood. There are chapters of existing organizations on a national level. Perhaps there is none in your small town, but you can participate on a county or state level. If you can't travel or leave your partner, participate at home. Letter writing is a start. E-mail is an avenue to explore. You can write or e-mail most elected officials. Enough letters on a hot issue get attention. Many organizations distribute letters to their members to sign and send. This insures a deluge of correspondence. A bombardment of letters may not get action, but does get attention which could be an incentive for eventual action.

You do not have to limit yourself to an advocating organization. Try to influence your fellow church members. Go to local clergymen even if you don't belong to a religious group, to ask for help in advertising your need and your cause. Become a member or better yet, an activist in a local public policy group. You can look for lay groups that wish to promote better conditions for handicapped people. Become a nudge to friends and relatives about your cause.

Present programs need to be preserved, as well as new ones entering the field. City and state budgets are subject to cutbacks all the time. Mayors and governors are always trying to keep down costs. You may see the importance of the need, but it seems as though the needy are the first to experience the tightening belt. Social service programs are the ones first affected. Many of the recipients of these programs are weak and may not even vote. Notice that elderly groups are most proactive when it comes to cutbacks or new legislation. The elderly are a formidable voting bloc, and assemblymen, senators, and governors are respectful of their demands, whether they intend to back them or not. Many of the older people are so active that the politicians know them personally.

Naomi was a ninety-plus lady who had been an activist since she was old enough to march. She was a member of a senior center and on the mayor's board of advisors on the issues of older people. She trudged to the state capital whenever an old benefit would be threatened or a new one proposed. She forced her way into the governor's office even though he did not have an open-door policy. Obviously, accosting a very old lady and her cane was not easy for young, able-bodied sentries. The governor knew her by name and whether or not he intended to espouse her cause, listened attentively. Naomi reached her 100th birthday and still accompanied protesting groups to the state capital and Washington. She died at 103, exhorting her great-grandchildren to carry on her job.

We can't all be that active, but we can be dedicated to an issue and participate in whatever way we can to help make changes. Keep informed. Even if you are housebound, pay close attention to newspapers, television, radio, and if you have a computer, go to the Internet. Remember that anything good or bad that affects the poor, the weak, the sick, or needy population of any kind may be of significance to you and your partner's disability. Medical issues, access to education, transportation, any of these topics may eventually affect you both. Watch how the groups or individuals oppose new incentives, or watch how advocates resist downsizing of old and approach the debate. Learn not only the methods they use, but also note the people they try to involve. Jot down phone numbers of interest groups that follow current issues applying to the needy, as well as those exposing injustices. Observe through these TV shows how citizens like you go about trying to make changes. I am not suggesting that you charge ahead like a crusader or Joan of Arc – only that you watch, listen, and absorb. Sooner or later, you will find your niche in advocacy.

The Constitution guarantees equal rights to all. It does not say equal rights to everyone except the deaf, the blind, or the lame. They are entitled to be able to take public transportation, get an education, receive training in a career of interest, attend public performances, and have adequate medical services, housing, food, and every other benefit available to the hale and hardy.

Eric was unable to ambulate without his wheelchair. He went with his wife Emily intending to cast his vote in a hotly contested presidential election. He had strong feelings about his candidate and wanted his voice heard. Their voting location was in the basement of a school. When they reached the polls and went to the elevator, they found an out of order sign. Eric was furious and Emily tried to find out if there was any other access to the voting booths. There was not. The poll officials had no solution. The time limit to submit absentee ballots was long past, and there was no other way to submit a paper ballot. Emily voted and they returned home angry and dejected. Eric, an intelligent man who had closely watched the campaign, had been disenfranchised because of his physical inability to manage a flight of stairs. Not providing him access to vote was not only unfair, but also illegal. However, the polling officials saw it only as a minor inconvenience for a small group of people. The apologies were forthcoming but did not appease Eric's outrage.

The government grants you your rights and also insures you the right exercise them. You may say, at this point, "What do you want from me? I am overburdened and you are urging me to do more? Let someone else fight for rights. I am too weary." Your point is well taken, but who is the "someone else"? Will the "someone else" be sensitive to your problems? Maybe he will or maybe he will not. But maybe despite all his fervor and incentives, he is unable to realize how frustrated you are, and how desperate you are for better, affordable services. He has not walked in your shoes. You have that edge on everybody else, and a vested interest in achieving your goals.

Dreams of a better life can spur you on. Please dream. Please act. Not for me or the greater good, but for yourself.

Chapter 16

Journey's End

My purpose in writing this book is to inspire you to develop techniques that will lighten your care giving responsibilities. If you succeed and manage to have some time for yourself, your focus shifts to "what now". At that moment, you may not have a clue. You have been totally involved in caregiving for a long time. You have to absorb the idea of an ongoing respite, the chance to add something new to your life. Give it time. Relax for a while. Thinking about yourself and the opportunity to broaden your horizons is a new, perhaps scary experience. You should think of the concept of "what's good for me" until it becomes a familiar refrain. Remember, the purpose of this precious free time is *not* to do laundry or other chores just because no one will interrupt you. The purpose of freeing up this time has always been to create the possibility of expanding your options.

What does pique your curiosity? What have you secretly dreamed of doing? Don't worry if it seems unusual or bizarre. Your interests are peculiar to you and not up for criticism. Your time alone doesn't have to be filled with "meaningful experiences" unless that's what you want. This time is significant as long as you are benefiting yourself. You can take a yoga class, swim, go to the beauty parlor, treat yourself to a massage, or sit in a coffee shop chatting with a friend. These activities do not waste precious time, not if you enjoy what you are doing and/or it helps you relax and regroup. By the same token, if you decide you want to take esoteric courses, prepare for part-time work at home, or a plan a future career, do so now. Being released from some of your caregiving chores means you are free to utilize that precious time to pamper yourself, fulfill intellectual desires, or prepare for a future job. The choice is yours.

At first, this will not be easy for you. You most likely will feel guilty about enjoying yourself, worry about how your partner is getting along without you, or be afraid that the stove will blow up. You have no reason to worry about what might happen and certainly no reason to feel guilty. The world will not collapse in your absence. You are entitled to free time and that time need not be riddled with "what ifs." Maybe you can't stop worrying just like that, but try to put your domestic concerns on the back burner when you are out. After all, you are only taking an hour off or a whole afternoon or even an entire day. You are not running off to join the circus. You will be going back home when your free time is over. All your worries will be waiting for you when you return. Let your helper worry while you are out. Trust her and don't be calling on the cell phone every ten minutes. Give her your cell phone number for a real emergency, then relax and go ahead with doing the "what I want for me" campaign.

If you are able to reassess your time to take care of your "wants," then all this looking into your inner self has not been in vain. Even if you can't get the free time right now, at least you can go about your chores with more understanding of yourself and your partner. Think of yourself positively and try to laugh a lot. Laughter is very important. Your everyday life is not a joke. However, try to joke about something. Make wisecracks to people. See if you can invoke smiles instead of pity. You don't have to be a comedy star to make yourself and those around you laugh. You may find that being funny takes some of the bite out of your daily life. Your circumstances are tragic but you mourning or sighing won't make it better. Laughter does not change a bad situation but at it can lighten your mood.

I conceived this book in hopes it could help you develop a new perspective. I have tried to propose some principles and ideas to make your life easier. However, changes will come about only if you initiate them. This is only a guide. Hopefully, you can draw a new road map for your journey and travel less bumpy roads. Delving into yourself to understand your motives in a different way was not easy for you. Soul-searching and self-analysis is a painful process. You should be commended for engaging in the task. It was worth the pain only if you have a better sense of what makes you tick. It was worth the pain if you can stop feeling so helpless. Even if you can't unshackle your life, you have the potential to liberate your spirit! Go for it!

www.ingramcontent.com/pod-product-compliance
Lightning Source LLC
Chambersburg PA
CBHW021952170526
45157CB00003B/954